OXFORD MEDICAL PUBLICATIONS

PATHOLOGY OF PERIODONTAL DISEASE

Pathology of Periodontal Disease

•

DAVID M. WILLIAMS

*The London Hospital Medical College, London, UK
and
College of Dentistry, University of Iowa, USA*

FRANCIS J. HUGHES

The London Hospital Medical College, London, UK

EDWARD W. ODELL

*United Medical and Dental Schools,
Guy's Hospital, London, UK*

AND

PAULA M. FARTHING

The London Hospital Medical College, London, UK

Oxford   New York   Tokyo

OXFORD UNIVERSITY PRESS

Oxford University Press, Walton Street, Oxford OX2 6DP

Oxford New York
Athens Auckland Bangkok Bogota Bombay
Buenos Aires Calcutta Cape Town Dar es Salaam
Delhi Florence Hong Kong Istanbul Karachi
Kuala Lumpur Madras Madrid Melbourne
Mexico City Nairobi Paris Singapore
Taipei Tokyo Toronto

and associated companies in
Berlin Ibadan

Oxford is a trade mark of Oxford University Press

Published in the United States by
Oxford University Press Inc., New York

First published 1992
Reprinted 1995, 1996

A catalogue record for this book is available from the British Library

Library of Congress Cataloging in Publication Data
Pathology of periodontal disease / David M. Williams . . . [et al.].
(Oxford medical publications)
Includes bibliographical references and index.
1. Periodontal disease.   I. Williams, David M. (David Michael)
II. Series.
[DNLM: 1. Periodontal Diseases.   WU 240 P297]
RK361P29   1992   617.6'32—dc20   91–27234
ISBN 0 19 262120 3

Printed in Hong Kong

PREFACE

Research into the pathological processes involved in periodontal disease has led to significant advances in our understanding of the condition in the last 20 years. However, whilst the results of this work are known to those engaged in research, they have not been disseminated widely and in straightforward terms to the dental profession at large. Our purpose in writing this book has been to distil an enormous body of detailed, careful research into a coherent logical account of periodontal disease.

The book was written in the first place with undergraduate dental students in mind, but we hope that it will also be useful to those engaged on M.Sc. courses and other postgraduate studies; to those preparing for their final Fellowship Examinations of the Royal Colleges; and to general dental practitioners. These groups have been borne in mind throughout the book. We have, therefore, tried to present ideas in a clear-cut and unambiguous fashion. Where differing and possibly conflicting opinions exist, we have reflected this in the text, but have then generally favoured one point of view over others. No doubt there will be those among our readers who will disagree with the stance we have sometimes taken. Given the level of vigorous debate which takes place among research workers, it would be surprising if it were otherwise.

We have quite deliberately not included exhaustive references. To do so would have interrupted the argument, and is not appropriate in a book of this kind. However, we have included a carefully selected, but deliberately short, reading list after each chapter. Some of the issues which are discussed in the book are not easily grasped on first encounter. For this reason we have made frequent use of diagrams and tables to summarize the text, and a list of conclusions is included at the end of each chapter.

Writing this book has been an intellectually challenging exercise and we have benefited enormously from the expert contributions of Dr Haroun Shah and Dr Ros Hopps who joined the group in writing Chapter 4 and Chapter 6.

ACKNOWLEDGEMENTS

We are grateful to our colleagues for their helpful and constructive comments in the writing of this book. In particular, we acknowledge the contribution of Dr Haroun Shah for his assistance in Chapter 4 and Dr Ros Hopps for her assistance with Chapter 6. We also wish to thank Dr Alan Saxton of Unilever Dental Research for permission to reproduce the scanning electron micrographs of dental plaque in Chapter 4, and Drs John and Deborah Greenspan and Dr Jim Winkler from the University of California, San Francisco, for the illustrations of HIV-associated periodontal disease in Chapter 7.

We would like to acknowledge the secretarial assistance of Mrs Christine Hall for her cheerful re-typing of several of the chapters in this book. The expert photographic assistance of Mr Michael Kelly is also acknowledged with gratitude.

Finally, we must express our thanks to our respective families and partners for their forbearance and support whilst we have been engaged in writing this book.

CONTENTS

1 The nature of periodontal disease

1.1 Introduction

Periodontal disease is a major problem for the oral health worker. It is the result of the accumulation of dental plaque at the marginal gingivae leading to inflammation of the periodontal tissues. Periodontal disease is prevalent in most human populations and results in significant morbidity, with premature tooth loss in severely affected individuals. Much research has been carried out into the epidemiology, aetiology, prevention, and clinical management of periodontal disease, and this has resulted in a significant increase in our understanding of the condition. In this chapter, the nature of periodontal disease will be considered in order to set the scene for the more detailed consideration of its pathogenesis in subsequent chapters. Following a general introduction to gingivitis and periodontitis, the different recognized types of periodontal disease are described, followed by a discussion of the aetiology of periodontal disease, consideration of its natural history, and an introduction to current concepts in the progression of the disease.

Traditionally, periodontal disease has been divided into gingivitis and periodontitis, depending on whether destruction of the periodontal attachment has occurred, and into acute or chronic conditions. In most cases periodontal disease is a chronic condition which persists for many years.

1.1.1 Gingivitis

Chronic gingivitis is defined as inflammation of the marginal gingival tissues due to the accumulation of dental plaque and is characterized clinically by redness, swelling, and bleeding of the tissues. The underlying periodontal ligament and alveolar bone are not involved and the epithelial attachment does not extend apically beyond its normal postition at the amelo-cemental junction. The condition is usually painless and is fully reversible following treatment. Gingival swelling due to inflammation may result in an increased probing depth without attachment loss. This is known as a false pocket. Many epidemiological studies have reported that chronic gingivitis is present in more than 95 per cent of the adult population. Some workers have questioned whether gingivitis can be considered a disease at all, because it is a normal response to the colonization of the teeth by the commensal oral flora and it does not result in any significant damage to the host. The World Health Organization has defined health as 'a state of complete physical and mental well-being' and it is difficult to see how the presence of painless inflammation at the gingival margins detracts seriously from this state. However, periodontitis is invariably associated with gingival inflammation and gingivitis appears to be a prerequisite for the development of periodontitis, although this is difficult to prove directly.

1.1.2 Periodontitis

Chronic periodontitis is defined as plaque-induced inflammation of the periodontal tissues which has resulted in destruction of the periodontal ligament, loss of crestal alveolar bone, and apical migration of the epithelial attachment (junctional epithelium). These processes are usually referred to collectively as loss of attachment. Periodontitis is characterized by the presence of inflammation at the marginal gingivae, together with loss of attachment, which normally results in the formation of a periodontal pocket and is often referred to as destructive periodontal disease. A periodontal pocket is a 'pathologically-deep-ened gingival crevice' characterized by the migration of junctional epithelium on to the root surface. Radiographically it is identified by loss of bone from the alveolar crest. Like chronic gingivitis, chronic periodontitis is usually painless. Adequate treatment of a site affected by periodontitis results in the resolution of inflammation and reduction in pocket depth, but this is not usually asssociated with the regeneration of lost periodontal ligament and crestal alveolar bone. In this sense, the tissue destruction seen in periodontitis is irreversible.

1.2 Types of periodontal disease

It is possible to recognize a number of different types of periodontal disease on the basis of clinical and pathological criteria, which include the extent of periodontal destruction, age of onset and severity of disease, distribution of lesions, the microflora involved, and variations in host responses. A classification of the distinct types of periodontal disease which are recognized, based on the report of the World Workshop in Periodontology in 1988, is shown in Table 1.1.

Table 1.1　Classification of periodontal disease

Gingivitis
　Childhood gingivitis
　Chronic (adult) gingivitis
　Acute necrotizing ulcerative gingivitis

Periodontitis
　Adult periodontitis
　Possible subgroups:　High risk
　　　　　　　　　　　Normal risk
　　　　　　　　　　　Refractory periodontitis

　Early onset periodontitis
　　Localized juvenile periodontitis
　　Rapidly progressive periodontitis
　　Pre-pubertal periodontitis
　Subgroups:　Localized
　　　　　　　Generalized

Periodontal disease associated with systemic factors
　Described in Table 1.5

1.2.1 Gingivitis

Childhood gingivitis

Most children are not affected by destructive periodontal disease, despite the fact that their plaque control is rarely optimal. Gingivitis is seldom seen before the age of six years, but its prevalence increases gradually until puberty, when over 90 per cent of children are affected. The characteristic clinical feature of childhood gingivitis is that it does not appear to progress to periodontitis. Histological studies have also shown that the inflammatory infiltrate seen in childhood gingivitis differs from that seen in adult gingivitis (see Chapter 3).

Chronic (adult) gingivitis

Chronic gingivitis associated with plaque accumulation is almost universally prevalent in the adult population, but wide individual variations in the clinical signs of gingivitis are seen. These include different amounts of gingival bleeding, swelling, and redness. Although some of the most prominent differences are due to plaque levels and secondary modifying factors (see p. 7 and p. 9), it is clear that clinical variations may also result from the presence of different micro-organisms in the plaque, and different sensitivities to plaque accumulation between individuals. Gingivitis may persist unchanged for many years, or it may result in the development of periodontitis.

Acute necrotizing ulcerative gingivitis

Acute necrotizing ulcerative gingivitis (ANUG) is a specific condition which mainly affects young adults with poor oral hygiene and other predisposing factors, such as a defective host response. It is characterized by the acute onset of painful, severely inflamed gingivae, with 'punched out' ulcers at the gingival margins, particularly affecting the inter-dental papillae, and a characteristic halitosis or 'foetor oris'. The condition may resolve after a few days, but is prone to recur in the absence of treatment. In recent years, ANUG has almost disappeared in many Western populations. A similar though more chronic condition resembling ANUG has recently been described in patients infected with the human immunodeficiency virus (HIV) and suffering from the acquired immune deficiency syndrome (AIDS). ANUG and HIV-related periodontal disease are considered in more detail in Chapter 7.

1.2.2 Adult periodontitis

Adult periodontitis (chronic periodontitis) is the common form of periodontitis seen in the adult population. It is characterized by inflammation and loss of periodontal attachment which usually starts after the age of 30 years and may affect any or all of the teeth. Adult periodontitis shows considerable inter-subject variation in its behaviour. Research suggests that most patients suffering from adult periodontitis have a relatively low risk of tooth loss, but approximately 10 per cent of patients may develop a more rapidly progressing form of the disease. Recently, a further small subgroup of patients with adult periodontitis has been proposed, in whom normal treatment procedures are ineffective in halting the progress of the disease. This condition has been referred to as 'refractory periodontitis', but whether it can be regarded as a specific entity remains a matter of conjecture.

Although adult periodontitis is a chronic disease, acute exacerbations are sometimes seen, with the formation of lateral periodontal abscesses. These are characterized by an accumulation of pus in the periodontal pocket, with pain and swelling. An untreated abscess will eventually drain into the oral cavity, either through the mouth of the pocket at the gingival margin or through a sinus. When this happens, a chronic abscess may develop, resulting in persistent pus formation and discharge. It is not clear why abscesses develop, but they may result from changes in the subgingival flora, true bacterial invasion of the tissues (which occurs following instrumentation of the pocket), or because the mouth of the pocket becomes blocked.

1.2.3 Early onset periodontitis

A few patients are unusually susceptible to periodontal breakdown and present with conditions distinct from those seen in adult periodontitis. These conditions develop in young people and are characterized by the onset and rapid progression of periodontal disease, giving rise to the term 'early onset periodontitis'. It is estimated that around one per cent of the population may be affected by early onset periodontitis, which may present as localized juvenile periodontitis (LJP), rapidly progressive periodontitis, or pre-pubertal periodontitis. These conditions are described briefly below, and in more detail in Chapter 7.

Localized juvenile periodontitis (LJP)

Localized juvenile periodontitis is characterized by severe periodontal breakdown localized to the permanent first molar and incisor teeth, with onset seen around puberty. The gingival tissues often appear relatively uninflamed and plaque accumulation is not prominent. Overall it has a prevalence of about 0.1 per cent of the population in Western countries, although it is more common in Afro-Carribean populations. It has been reported to affect females more than males and there appears to be a familial basis in at least some instances. Microbiological studies have indicated that the bacterium *Actinobacillus actinomycetemcomitans* may have an important aetiological role.

Rapidly progressive periodontitis (RPP)

Rapidly progressive periodontitis has similarities to LJP, but severe periodontal breakdown tends to be more generalized, affecting any teeth, and the age of onset is usually after about 20 years of age. During more acute stages, the gingivae have been reported to be unusually red and sore and, once again, only low levels of plaque accumulation may be seen. Less is known about the epidemiology of this condition than about LJP, although it appears to be more common and it may have a familial tendency. *A. actinomycetemcomitans* appears to be a less prominent constituent of the microflora of RPP when compared to LJP, but high levels of *Porphyromonas gingivalis* have been found.

Pre-pubertal periodontitis

This condition is extremely rare and is characterized by severe periodontal breakdown in the deciduous dentition. It has been reported in generalized and localized forms, and usually responds poorly to even the most intensive treatment. The deciduous dentition may also be affected by periodontal breakdown in a few unusual systemic diseases, discussed on pp. 115–17.

1.2.4 Periodontal disease associated with systemic factors

In addition to the types of periodontal disease discussed above, a number of systemic factors may act to modify the host response to plaque accumulation, resulting in distinct and well recognized forms of periodontal disease, such as pregnancy gingivitis and drug-induced gingival hyperplasia. The role of systemic factors in the aetiology of periodontal disease will be considered on pp. 6–9.

1.2.5 Other diseases of the periodontal tissues

Although periodontal disease is caused by the accumulation of dental plaque, the periodontal tissues may also be affected in a number of other conditions which are not due primarily to plaque accumulation and are not, therefore, types of periodontal disease. These conditions include specific infections such as acute herpetic gingivo-stomatitis, muco-cutaneous conditions such as lichen planus, benign mucous membrane pemphigoid, and pemphigus vulgaris, and neoplasms such as squamous cell carcinoma. A list of some of these conditions is given in Table 1.2. Although they are much less common than periodontal disease, it is important for the clinician to recognize that they may produce similar signs and symptoms. Furthermore, it is common for any of these conditions to present with superimposed periodontal disease. A detailed account of these diseases is beyond the scope of this book and readers are referred to standard texts in oral medicine and oral pathology for their further consideration.

Table 1.2   Examples of diseases which may affect the periodontal tissues and are not due primarily to plaque accumulation

Type of condition	Clinical features
Traumatic	
Mechanical, chemical, or thermal trauma	Ulceration
Infectious	
Herpetic gingivo-stomatitis	Erythema; ulceration
Candidiasis	Erythema; white plaques
Immunological muco-cutaneous disease	
Lichen planus	Desquamative gingivitis; white striae
Pemphigus	Desquamative gingivitis
Benign mucous membrane pemphigoid	Desquamative gingivitis
Major aphthous ulceration	Ulceration
Neoplastic	
Squamous cell carcinoma	Swelling; ulceration; bone loss
Leukaemias	Gingival swelling; ulceration
Multiple myeloma	Destruction of alveolar bone
Histiocytosis X/eosinophilic granuloma	Destruction of alveolar bone
Benign tumours	Swelling
Granulomatous	
Crohn's Disease	Gingival hyperplasia
Sarcoidosis	Gingival hyperplasia
Wegener's granulomatosis	Gingival hyperplasia
Intoxication	
Heavy metal poisoning (e.g. Hg, Pb, Bi)	Pigmentation of gingival tissues
Hereditary	
Hereditary gingival fibromatosis	Gingival hyperplasia

1.3 The aetiology of periodontal disease

1.3.1 Primary and secondary factors

Bacterial plaque is the primary aetiological factor in periodontal disease and the disease will not occur in the absence of plaque. There is overwhelming evidence to support this view, including epidemiological data, clinical studies which have investigated the effects of plaque accumulation and its removal, and pathological, microbiological, and immunological data. This evidence is considered further in Chapter 4. In addition, a number of well recognized factors may influence or modify the nature of periodontal disease, although they do not in themselves cause the disease. These factors are often referred to as secondary factors and can be divided into those which act locally in the oral environment and those which act via a systemic route (Table 1.3).

Table 1.3 Aetiology of periodontal disease

Primary factor	Secondary factors	
Dental plaque	Local:	plaque traps
		lack of saliva
		occlusal trauma
	Systemic:	genetic
		infections
		hormonal
		drug-induced
		haematological
		nutritional

1.3.2 Local secondary factors

Most local secondary factors are mechanical plaque traps, promoting plaque accumulation at specific sites (Table 1.4). Such factors include the presence of calculus, carious cavities, overhanging margins of restorations, and partial dentures. The effect of these factors is to increase the amount of plaque at a specific site, but this in turn may alter the proportions of different bacterial species. Anatomical variations also act as secondary factors in periodontal disease. For example, the presence of a canine fossa may predispose to plaque accumulation on the mesial surface of upper first premolars. Persistent mouth-breathing results in a lack of saliva in the anterior regions of the mouth, due to drying. The hyperplastic gingivitis which results has been attributed to accelerated plaque accumulation resulting from the loss of the anti-bacterial

Table 1.4 Some local secondary aetiological factors which may predispose to periodontal disease

Mechanical plaque traps
  Calculus
  Carious cavities
  Margins of restorations
  Partial dentures and other intra-oral appliances
  Crowding and malocclusions
  Anatomical variations of tooth morphology

Decreased anti-bacterial actions of saliva
  Mouthbreathing
  Xerostomia

Occlusal trauma
  Unknown mechanism

Table 1.5   Effects of some systemic secondary factors on periodontal disease

Conditions which cause gingival hyperplasia

Hormonal changes
Pregnancy; contraceptive pill; puberty	Increased progesterone levels cause vascular changes in the gingival tissues. This results in a hyperplastic, haemorrhagic gingivitis. Epulis formation may also occur. Condition will resolve with meticulous plaque control

Drug induced
Phenytoin; cyclosporin A; nifedipine	Action of the drug or its metabolites on fibroblasts results in gingival hyperplasia. Characterized by pink fibrous gingival swellings. Hyperplasia can be reduced by adequate plaque control

Defects in host defences resulting in accelerated periodontal breakdown

Hormonal
Insulin-dependent diabetes mellitus	Increased periodontal destruction and susceptibility to periodontal abscesses have been reported. Effect seen mainly in poorly controlled or undiagnosed diabetics. Possibly due to impaired neutrophil function, although other changes could be responsible

HIV infection
	Chronic necrotising ulcerative gingivitis, severe destructive periodontitis; erythematous gingivitis. See Chapter 7 for a more detailed discussion

Neutrophil defects
Cyclic neutropaenia; other neutropaenias	Severe destructive periodontitis is a marked feature of all chronic neutropaenic states
Leukaemias	Severe destructive periodontitis, associated with neutropaenia. In addition, gingival swelling may be seen, due to the accumulation of large numbers of leukaemic cells in the gingival tissues

Genetic
Down's syndrome	Severe destructive periodontitis seen in young adult patients. Does not appear to be solely the result of poor plaque control. Believed to be due to impaired neutrophil function
Papillon–Lefèvre syndrome	Very rare syndrome where pre-pubertal periodontitis is seen in association with palmar–plantar keratosis (thickening of the skin on the palms of the hands and soles of the feet). Associated with neutrophil defects
Chediak–Higashi syndrome	Rare syndrome involving lysosomal defects in many cell types, notably neutrophils, and associated with severe infections including destructive periodontitis

Connective tissue defects resulting in accelerated periodontal breakdown

Nutritional
Ascorbic acid deficiency (scurvy)	Haemorrhagic gingivitis and increased periodontal destruction associated with defective collagen synthesis and vascular fragility. Very rare in developed countries
Kwashiorkor (protein deficiency)	Severe malnutrition seen almost exclusively in Africa, resulting in alterations in connective tissue regulation and disruption of many other homeostatic mechanisms. ANUG can be severe and progress to cancrum oris, where massive necrosis results from the spread of infection from the gingivae to other oro-facial tissues

Genetic
Hypophosphatasia	Vitamin D-resistant rickets leading to skeletal changes similar to those of dietary rickets. Almost complete absence of cementum formation results in rapid periodontal breakdown and early loss of the deciduous dentition
Ehlers–Danlos syndrome	Disorder of collagen metabolism. Rapid periodontal breakdown is a feature of one variant of this condition

and lubricating actions of saliva. Patients who suffer from a dry mouth may also have increased gingivitis for the same reason. The antibacterial actions of saliva are discussed in Chapter 5.

The significance of occlusal trauma as an aetiological factor in periodontal disease has been the subject of much controversy. Although the excessive occlusal loading of teeth will result in a widening of the periodontal ligament and increased mobility, this is not associated with the formation of periodontal pockets and appears to be an adaptive change of the supporting structures of the teeth. A number of animal studies where teeth have been subjected to excessive occlusal forces have demonstrated that occlusal trauma will not initiate periodontal breakdown, even in the presence of bacterial plaque. However, it is believed that such forces might exacerbate breakdown at an already active site, although the mechanism by which this occurs is not fully understood.

1.3.3 Systemic secondary factors

Systemic factors act in a number of ways to increase or modify periodontal disease caused by plaque accumulation. Although these factors are often classified using a surgical sieve as shown in Table 1.3, they may also be divided into those which cause gingival hyperplasia, those which are associated with impaired host defences and result in increased periodontal destruction, and a few rare connective tissue disorders which can result in increased periodontal destruction (see Table 1.5).

The most commonly encountered systemic factor is the changing level of hormones seen in pregnancy. Increased progesterone secretion results in alterations in the gingival vasculature and in the inflammatory response. In the presence of plaque, these lead to the characteristic features of pregnancy gingivitis, which include an unusually severe haemorrhagic gingivitis with prominent gingival hyperplasia. At times, the hyperplasia may result in a gross localized swelling – the pregnancy epulis (pyogenic granuloma of pregnancy). Similar features may also be seen in girls during puberty and in those who take the contraceptive pill, although these conditions are usually less severe than in pregnancy.

Certain medications, such as the anticonvulsant drug phenytoin, may give rise to gingival hyperplasia. It is believed that a metabolite of phenytoin has a stimulatory effect on gingival fibroblasts, giving rise to the characteristic pink, fibrous gingival hyperplasia. Similar changes are also seen in patients taking the immunosuppressive drug cyclosporin A, which is widely used to prevent graft rejection following organ transplant, and the calcium channel blocker nifedipine, which is a coronary artery vasodilator.

Severe periodontal breakdown is associated with conditions in which neutrophil defects occur, and this is discussed further in Chapter 5. Patients who suffer from insulin-dependent diabetes mellitus have been reported to show increased periodontal breakdown associated with impaired neutrophil function, but the evidence for this is controversial. The most recent evidence suggests that only those with undiagnosed or poorly controlled diabetes may be particularly susceptible to increased periodontal disease.

1.4 The natural history of periodontal disease

Although periodontal disease usually affects many teeth in the same mouth, this does not mean that all areas are equally affected by the disease or behave in exactly the same manner. Consequently, the disease is often investigated by looking at individual *sites* within the mouth. Sites are defined as those parts of the crevice measured with a periodontal probe at standard positions, usually mesio-buccal, mid-buccal, disto-buccal, mesio-lingual or mesio-palatal, mid-lingual, and disto-lingual.

Theoretically, there could be three different outcomes of disease at any given site:

- the persistence of inflammation without further loss of attachment – *stable or 'quiescent' lesion*

- continued loss of periodontal attachment – *disease progression or 'active' disease*

- healing – *resolution*

The presence of inflammation does not necessarily indicate progressive disease. Indeed, at present, there is no way of establishing whether a periodontal lesion is active or quiescent at any given time. Complete resolution of a lesion appears to be a very unusual event unless adequate plaque control measures are introduced, and thus the amount of attachment loss at a given site represents the cumulative effects of previous episodes of periodontal breakdown. These factors make it difficult to investigate accurately the progression of periodontal disease, but in recent years there has been considerable progress in overcoming these problems.

1.4.1 The investigation of disease progression

Cross-sectional studies

Investigations into the epidemiology and progression of periodontal disease may be divided into two basic types, cross-sectional and longitudinal studies. In cross-sectional studies, a number of different individuals are examined at a single point in time to determine the presence and severity of the disease. For example,

Subject	Age	Mean attachment loss
A	25	2.0
B	30	1.3
C	30	8.2
D	33	3.2
E	40	5.0
F	43	3.8
G	47	6.0
H	50	4.0
I	56	6.0
J	56	8.1
K	60	10.1
L	65	8.0
M	68	8.7
N	60	2.1

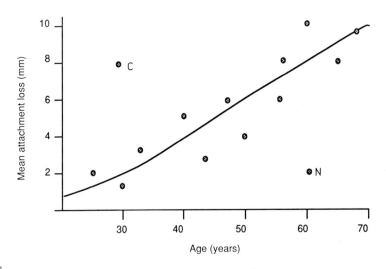

Fig. 1.1 Hypothetical cross-sectional data of mean attachment loss in 14 subjects. The average rate of attachment loss (solid line) is approximately 2 mm every 10 years, but it is clear that there is considerable inter-subject variation. Subject C appears to be highly susceptible to periodontal breakdown. Subject N appears to be relatively resistant to breakdown.

when examining the progression of periodontal disease in the population, the amount of attachment loss seen in different subjects is plotted against their age to determine the overall progression of disease (see Fig. 1.1). These studies can be completed relatively quickly and are not dependent on maintaining contact with individual subjects over a long period of time. Their main disadvantage is that, because they only measure disease at a single point in time, it is only possible to deduce general trends in the progression of disease within the population. Such studies give no information about how the disease is likely to behave in individual patients. For example, in the data shown in Fig. 1.1, the results appear to suggest that the mean pocket depth found in 30-year-old subjects will increase by 2 mm in the next ten years. However, in the absence of information about the rate of disease progression, this conclusion does not apply to specific individuals and such studies cannot be used to determine the rate of disease progression.

Longitudinal studies

In order to study the progression of periodontal disease accurately, longitudinal studies are required, involving repeated examinations over a period of time. These have considerable advantages in determining patterns of disease progression, because they involve a direct measurement of the progression of disease in sites from *individual* subjects (see Fig. 1.2). Although longitudinal studies are greatly superior to cross-sectional studies for the investigation of disease progression, they do have some potential problems, which need to be overcome if they are to give useful results. One disadvantage is that they are more time-consuming than cross-sectional studies and it takes a longer time to obtain useful results. In practice, it is extremely difficult to follow the same subjects over a lifetime's experience of periodontal disease. Furthermore, during any longitudinal study a number of subjects will be lost, due to factors such as moving house or loss of cooperation. This raises the possibility that the results in the subjects who 'drop out' may have been different from the rest of the group, leading to a bias in the final results. Those subjects with the least interest in dental health and the worst periodontal disease may be those most likely to drop out from a study, so that the rate and extent of disease progression might be underestimated.

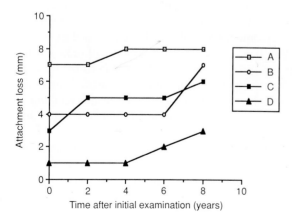

Time (years)	A	B	C	D
0	1	3	4	7
2	1	5	4	7
4	1	5	4	8
6	2	5	4	8
8	3	6	7	8

Fig. 1.2 Hypothetical longitudinal data showing the attachment loss at four different sites (A, B, C, D) in one patient at an initial examination and after periods of two, four, six, and eight years.

Clinical measurement of disease

In addition to the limitations of clinical studies which have been discussed, it can be extremely difficult to make accurate and reproducible measurements of the amount of periodontal disease present. A number of different methods have been described for determining the presence and severity of periodontal disease. Many of these use indices to assign scores to different levels of disease, recording, for example, the severity of gingival inflammation, amount of plaque present, and loss of attachment. It is vital to interpret the results of measurements correctly. For example, indices used to measure the severity of gingival bleeding should not be used to give an indication of the severity of periodontal breakdown present.

A major problem with most periodontal indices is that an average is taken of the results from the measurement of a number of teeth from a number of patients. Consequently, although such indices may give an overall measure of the amount of disease in a population, they may not accurately measure the progression of disease in individual subjects. To overcome this difficulty, most current longitudinal studies take repeated measurements of attachment loss at individual sites, and record these separately. Attachment loss is measured by periodontal probing from a fixed reference point, the amelo-cemental junction. Such measurements are referred to as clinical attachment levels. The measured clinical attachment level may vary according to a number of factors, such as the probing force used, the position and angulation of the probe, the presence of subgingival calculus, or the amount of inflammation present at a particular site. A number of techniques are used in clinical studies to improve the reliability of attachment level measurements. These include the construction of custom-built acrylic stents (guides), to ensure a constant positioning and angulation of the probe, and the use of constant-pressure probes. However, despite the application of these laborious techniques, there is still variation in probing measurements, and it is impossible to measure changes of less than 1mm in attachment level accurately within the margin of experimental error.

The other approach to measuring loss of attachment involves the use of radiographs. These have the disadvantage that a two-dimensional view is obtained of a three-dimensional structure, and it is inevitable that information is lost by this process. Furthermore, changes detected radiographically may not always truly reflect changes in attachment levels. Once again, there are considerable problems with the accuracy and reproducibility of radiographic techniques in measuring attachment loss. Variations in the positioning and angulation of films, X-ray exposure, and processing are examples of some of the sources of error. Attempts to overcome these problems have included the use of standardized or custom-built film holders and batch processing of radiographs. Recently, computerized image analysis systems have been able to record data from radiographs electronically. Using this technique it is possible to make accurate comparisons of radiographs of the same site taken at different times, and to identify small areas of bone loss occurring in the interval between taking the two films.

Despite the considerable difficulties involved with longitudinal studies, they have yielded much valuable information about the natural history of periodontal disease and have had an important impact on the understanding of the disease, its causes, and its management.

1.4.2 The progression of periodontal disease

Gradual destruction model of disease progression

Cross-sectional epidemiological studies in the United Kingdom, the United States of America, and elsewhere have investigated the relationship between increasing age and the severity of periodontal disease. These studies have all shown a broadly similar linear correlation between age and attachment loss, with a *mean* rate of periodontal destruction of approximately 0.1–0.2 mm per year, although there are wide individual variations. These data can be interpreted as indicating that periodontal breakdown proceeds in a slow, inexorable fashion unless it is adequately treated, and this concept has been termed the 'gradual destruction model' of disease progression, illustrated in Fig. 1.3.

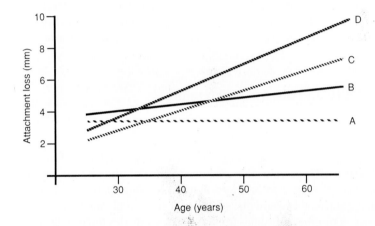

Fig. 1.3   Gradual destruction model of periodontal breakdown. The graph shows periodontal attachment loss at four sites (A, B, C, D). In the absence of adequate treatment the pockets slowly progress with time, although at different rates from each other.

Burst theory of periodontal breakdown

More recently, a number of longitudinal studies have recorded attachment loss at individual sites in different subjects. These have revealed that, despite the presence of inflammation, most sites showed no progression during the study period. Instead, attachment loss occurred in periods of rapid periodontal breakdown at only a few sites and was interspersed with long periods of quiescence. This theory of intermittent disease progression, where short periods of breakdown or active disease are interspersed with long periods of stability or quiescence, is termed the 'burst theory'. It has further been proposed that bursts might occur randomly in an individual throughout life, or there may be periods when bursts of periodontal breakdown in many sites are more likely. The terms 'random burst' and 'asynchronous multiple burst' respectively have been used to describe these concepts (Fig. 1.4).

The findings of these longitudinal studies have important implications for our understanding of the nature of periodontal disease. Firstly, the presence of plaque and inflammation at a site does not indicate that further periodontal breakdown is occurring or that it will occur at a later time. The most obvious example of this is seen in cases of gingivitis, which may persist for years without progressing to periodontitis. Secondly, the disease is 'site specific' and periodontal breakdown may affect different teeth in the same mouth at different rates. The concept of site specificity is of great clinical relevance, because it implies that diseased sites in a patient's mouth must be considered separately for diagnosis and treatment.

It is probable that much of the periodontal breakdown which is seen is the result of bursts of active disease. A burst of activity can account for more than

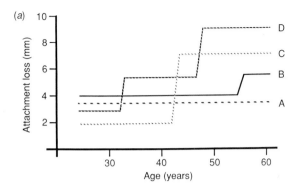

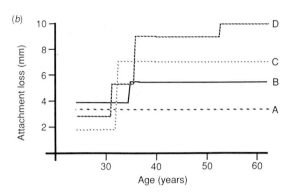

Fig. 1.4 Burst hypotheses of periodontal breakdown showing disease progression at four sites.

(a) Random burst model: periodontal disease progresses in short, randomly occurring bursts throughout adult life, interspersed with long periods of quiescence in between.

(b) Asynchronous multiple burst model: again, periodontal disease progresses in bursts, interspersed with periods of quiescence. However, most of the bursts are clustered during a short period of the patient's life – in this case between the ages of 30 and 35 years. Thus 'multiple bursts' occur from age 30–35, but they are not simultaneous (i.e. they are 'asynchronous').

3mm of attachment loss in a few weeks, and this may be particularly important as far as the long term periodontal support of affected teeth is concerned. However, because of the difficulty of measuring small changes in attachment level, studies of disease progression cannot exclude the possibility of some gradual destruction.

1.4.3 Susceptibility and disease progression

Susceptible and resistant patient groups

In addition to site specific variations in the behaviour of periodontal disease, it is apparent that different people show varying degrees of susceptibility to destructive periodontal disease. Thus, as well as the occurrence of attachment loss in a site-specific pattern, it may also be more marked in some patients than in others, even when quantifiable elements, such as the level of plaque control are taken into account. A number of studies from different countries have suggested that about 10 per cent of subjects appear to be at relatively high risk to destructive periodontal disease and experience severe periodontal destruction with rapid progression and tooth loss. About 80 per cent of the population are susceptible to periodontitis which progresses rather slowly and rarely results in total loss of the dentition. The remaining 10 per cent appear to be relatively resistant to destructive periodontitis, despite the continued presence of gingivitis. This division of the population into those at high risk, normal risk, or low risk of periodontal destruction may be an over simplification of the true picture, but there is presently a reasonable consensus for the existence of a 'high risk' group comprising around 10 per cent of the population.

Possible reasons for disease progression

Periodontal disease is the result of the interaction of bacteria and the factors derived from plaque with the host tissues. The destructive and protective mechanisms which operate in periodontal disease are normally considered to be in equilibrium, resulting in a stable or quiescent lesion. Bursts of periodontal breakdown may occur when this balance is upset, either because of an increase in destructive factors, or because of a decrease in the effectiveness of protective mechanisms. Variations in the destruction–protection balance may explain the variations in disease susceptibility which are seen. In principle, alterations in bacteria–host interactions may be due to alterations in either the bacterial flora or the host defences, and indeed there is evidence that both may be important in different situations. The destructive and protective mechanisms which may be important in periodontal disease are described in greater detail in later chapters.

The ability to identify the mechanisms likely to result in periodontal break-down might have important clinical implications. Firstly, it might be possible to identify and target high risk groups of patients for special care and management, and, secondly, it might be possible to determine more accurately the efficacy of treatment procedures. The reasons for the occurrence of periodontal destruction, the factors which may determine disease susceptibility, and the reasons for disease progression at different sites in the same patient are some of the most important questions in periodontology today.

1.5 Summary

1. Periodontal disease is a major public health problem and is found in all human populations. Its clinical presentations vary widely, from persistent gingivitis to severe destructive periodontitis.

2. On the basis of current clinical and pathological evidence, the forms of destructive periodontal disease which can be identified are adult periodontitis, localized juvenile periodontitis, rapidly progressive periodontitis, and pre-pubertal periodontitis.

3. The primary cause of periodontal disease is the accumulation of dental plaque at the gingival margins. A number of secondary aetiological factors may act locally or systemically to modify the disease state.

4. Despite the practical difficulties of monitoring the progression of periodontal disease, there is good evidence to show that the disease is episodic, with long periods of quiescence being interspersed with occasional bursts of rapid periodontal breakdown.

5. Periodontal disease is site-specific, affecting different sites in the same mouth to different extents. Different individuals show wide variations in their susceptibility to the disease.

6. Bursts of activity and variations in susceptibility may be due to imbalances between bacterial factors and host defences.

1.6 Further reading

Chilton, N. W. (1986). Conference on clinical trials in periodontal diseases. *J. Clin. Periodontol.* **13**, 336–549.
— *A series of papers covering many aspects of current thinking on the nature of periodontal disease, including some valuable discussions on the problems of conducting good clinical trials.*

Löe, H., Anerud, A., Boysen, H., and Smith, M. (1978). The natural history of periodontal disease in Man. *J. Periodontol.* **49**, 607–20.
— *Classic paper describing the epidemiology of periodontal disease, including the detection of high risk and low risk sub-populations.*

Page, R. C. and Schroeder, H. E. (1986). Periodontitis in man and other animals. (Karger, Basel).
— *Extensive discussion of the natural history of periodontal disease and classification of the various types of the disease.*

Papapanou, P. N., Wennström, J. L., and Gröndahl, K. (1989). A 10-year retrospective study of periodontal disease progression. *J. Clin. Periodontol.* **16**, 403–11.
— *Epidemiological study providing evidence for the existence of high risk and low risk groups.*

Pindborg, J. J. (1989). Manifestations of systemic disorders in the periodontium *and* Tumors originating from the periodontium. In *A Textbook of Clinical Periodontology*, 2nd edn. (ed. J. Lindhe). (Munksgaard, Copenhagen).
— *Discussion of systemic factors affecting periodontal disease, and other diseases which may affect the periodontal tissues.*

Socransky, S. S., Haffajee, A. D., Goodson, J. M., and Lindhe, J. (1984). New concepts of destructive periodontal disease. *J. Clin. Periodontol.* **11**, 21–32.
— *Classic description of burst theories in periodontal disease progression.*

2 The normal periodontium

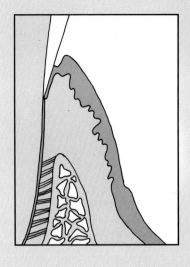

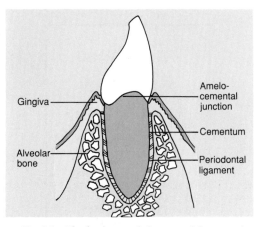

Fig. 2.1 The fundamental elements of the normal periodontium.

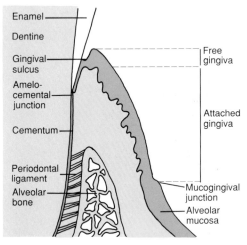

Fig. 2.2 The components of the coronal part of the normal periodontium.

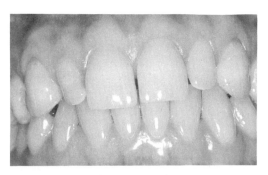

Fig. 2.3 Clinical photograph of the gingiva in perfect health. The attached gingiva is firm, pink, and stippled. The alveolar mucosa is thinner and appears red in colour. Small blood vessels can be seen beneath the surface of the alveolar mucosa.

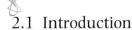

2.1 Introduction

Before discussing the processes and mechanisms involved in periodontal disease, it is important to establish a sound understanding of the structure of the normal periodontium. The basic elements and function are described in this section and on pp. 18–23 the gingiva is discussed in more detail. The periodontal ligament, alveolar bone, and cementum are dealt with on p. 23, p. 24, and p. 26 respectively. Although traditional representations of the periodontium tend to convey a rather static image, the tissues are in a continual state of turnover and this issue is addressed on pp. 26–9. This chapter is not intended as an exhaustive treatise on the periodontium, and a list of suggested further reading will be found at the end of the chapter.

The basic elements of the periodontium are the gingiva, periodontal ligament, alveolar bone, and cementum (Fig. 2.1). The function of the periodontium is to attach the teeth into the jaws and support them effectively during masticatory function. During the course of chewing, the loads which fall on the teeth cause small lateral and horizontal movements. A critical aspect of the structure of the periodontium is that it is able to accommodate these movements. The normal anatomical relationship of the elements of the periodontium in health are shown in Fig. 2.2.

2.2 The gingiva

The gingiva provides attachment between the oral mucous membrane and the dental hard tissues and protects the underlying periodontal tissues from invasion by the bacteria present in the oral cavity. In conditions of perfect health the gingiva appears pale pink, firm and stippled (Fig. 2.3) and is attached to the teeth at, or just above, the amelo-cemental junction (Fig. 2.2). The gingiva comprises fibrous connective tissue covered by epithelium and extends from the muco-gingival junction, where it abuts on the alveolar mucosa, to the tooth surface. The gingiva can be divided into two parts: the free gingiva and the attached gingiva.

The free gingiva is that portion of the gingiva coronal to the level of the epithelial attachment and includes the interdental papilla. In health this is at the amelo-cemental junction, but apical migration of the junctional epithelium occurs in disease (see Chapter 3), and the free gingiva will tend to move apically. The point at which the free gingiva abuts on the tooth above the epithelial attachment is called the gingival crevice or gingival sulcus. In conditions of absolute health this crevice is either absent or of minimal depth, but more commonly it is 1–2 mm in depth. The attached gingiva is bound down to bone in the form of a muco-periosteum. The mucosa in this area, together with the covering of the hard palate, is keratinized and is termed masticatory mucosa because it is directly exposed to the forces of mastication. The characteristic stippled appearance of the attached gingiva which is seen in health is attributable to the insertion of collagen fibres in the muco-periosteum into the underlying alveolar bone. The alveolar mucosa, which begins at the muco-gingival junction, is part of the lining mucosa of the mouth. It is brighter red in colour than the attached gingiva, because the overlying epithelium is thinner and non-keratinized, the connective tissue is more vascular, and it is not tightly bound down to bone.

2.2.1 The basic structure of oral epithelium

Oral epithelium is a stratified squamous epithelium and, like other similar epithelia, is composed of keratinocytes and non-keratinocytes or clear cells (Fig. 2.4). Keratinocytes make up the bulk of the cells, and in keratinizing sites, such as the oral gingival epithelium (Fig. 2.5), comprise the basal cell, prickle cell, granular cell, and keratinized layers. Cell division normally occurs only in the basal cell layer and the cells which arise from these divisions move gradually through the epithelium towards the surface, where they are shed (Fig. 2.4). During the course of this process the cells increase in size and their shape changes, so that by the time they reach the surface they have become flattened. These changes are accompanied by the synthesis of a number of cell products, the most conspicuous of which is keratin, which packs the cells in the keratinized layer and contributes to the mechanical toughness of the superficial layers. This process of maturation is termed differentiation. In non-keratinizing epithelia, such as the alveolar mucosa (Fig. 2.2), the changes in the keratinocytes are less marked than in keratinizing epithelia, and the granular cell and cornified layers are absent.

Fig. 2.4 The components of orthokeratinized stratified squamous epithelium. The changes in the keratinocytes associated with differentiation as they move towards the surface are represented. The non-keratinocyte or clear cell population, comprising Langerhans cells, melanocytes, lymphocytes, and Merkel cells, is also shown. These appearances are characteristic of masticatory mucosa, such as the attached gingiva or hard palate. In non-keratinized stratified squamous epithelia, typical of the lining mucosa (e.g. alveolar mucosa, buccal mucosa), the changes seen as cells move towards the surface are less marked. The granular cell and keratinized layers are replaced by the intermediate and surface layers and the keratinocyte nuclei are retained throughout the full thickness of the epithelium.

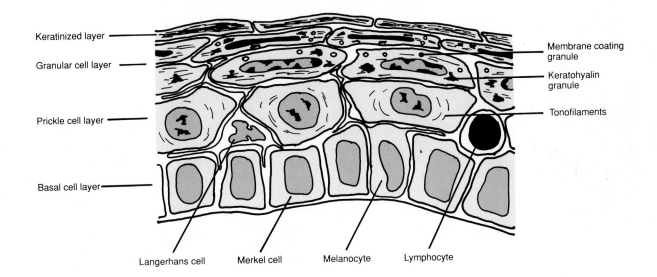

One of the most significant events during epithelial differentiation is the synthesis of membrane coating granules in the upper part of the prickle cell and granular cell layers (Fig. 2.4). These discharge their lipid contents into the intercellular space between the upper cell layers of both keratinized and non-keratinized epithelia, forming a barrier to the free permeability of water and water soluble substances. It should be emphasized that this is not an absolute barrier to permeability, and it varies significantly from site to site in the mouth. As will be discussed on p. 121, junctional epithelium (Figs 2.5–2.8) does not synthesize membrane coating granules and, as a consequence, lacks an effective permeability barrier.

The non-keratinocyte population of epithelium comprises melanocytes, lymphocytes, Langerhans cells, and Merkel cells. These cells are sometimes known

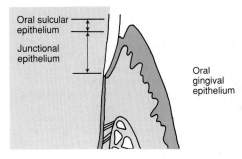

Fig. 2.5 The regions of the gingival epithelium.

collectively as clear cells, because of their appearance in routinely prepared microscope sections. Special techniques are required to demonstrate their true distribution and density. Although melanocytes and Merkel cells play no known active role in the inflammatory and immune reaction in periodontal disease (Chapter 5), lymphocytes and Langerhans cells are of major significance. Langerhans cells trap antigens on their long dendritic processes and present them to lymphocytes, either locally within the mucosa or following their migration to regional lymph nodes. This is one of the principal mechanisms by which immune responses are initiated and is important because it means that immune reactions can occur without the necessity for antigens to penetrate through the full thickness of the epithelium.

2.2.2 Gingival epithelium

The epithelium covering the gingiva can be divided into three regions which are illustrated diagrammatically in Fig. 2.5. The oral gingival epithelium is a stratified squamous epithelium which is normally orthokeratinized. The oral sulcular epithelium is that epithelium lining the gingival crevice or sulcus. It is non-keratinized and has a shallow rete-peg pattern. Although it faces the tooth surface, it does not participate directly in the epithelial attachment. The third type of epithelium is junctional epithelium.

2.2.3 Junctional epithelium

In health, the apical limit of the junctional epithelium is at or near the amelo-cemental junction. This epithelium forms the attachment of the gingiva to the tooth surface (the epithelial attachment), which it does by means of the hemidesmosomes which anchor the basal keratinocytes to the basement membrane (Fig. 2.6). The basement membrane at the interface between epithelium and connective tissue, which in health is relatively flat, continues up on to the enamel surface to the coronal limit of the junctional epithelium, and terminates in the base of the gingival crevice (Fig. 2.7). Under the light microscope, junctional epithelium can be distinguished from the oral sulcular epithelium because the orientation of the cells in the junctional epithelium is parallel to the tooth surface and it has wider intercellular spaces (Fig. 2.8). The presence of small numbers of neutrophils in the junctional epithelium is a well-recognized feature, even in

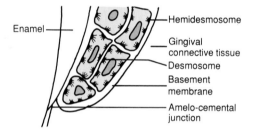

Fig. 2.6 The apical portion of the junctional epithelium. The basement membrane separates the junctional epithelium from the gingival connective tissue and then, at its most apical extent, near the amelo-cemental junction, it is reflected upwards on to the enamel surface. The epithelial cells, which themselves secrete important components of the basement membrane, are attached to it by hemidesmosomes.

Fig. 2.7 The coronal portion of the junctional epithelium. Attachment to the tooth surface occurs in the same way as in the apical portion (Fig. 2.6). Keratinocytes are shed from the junctional epithelium into the bottom of the gingival crevice and migrating neutrophils are also seen in this region, even in states of perfect gingival health. The keratinocyte population of the junctional epithelium is sustained by cell division in the lower part of the junctional epithelium, and there is a continuous movement of cells upwards into the gingival crevice. The cells in the junctional epithelium are orientated parallel to the tooth surface and have large intercellular spaces.

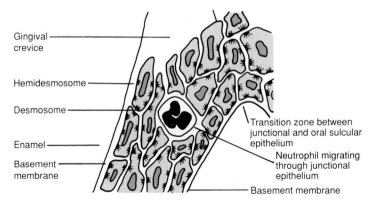

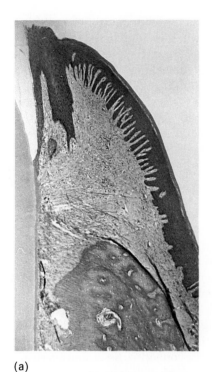

(a)

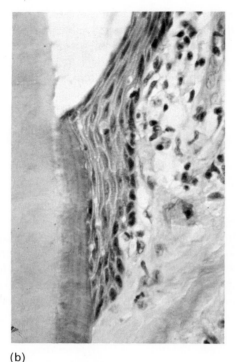

(b)

Fig. 2.8 The light microscope appearance of junctional epithelium.
Fig. 2.8(a) is a low-power view of the area shown diagrammatically in Fig. 2.2. The specimen has been demineralized, so that the junctional epithelium is seen abutting on the enamel space. There is no measurable gingival crevice in this section, so that the zone of the oral sulcular epithelium is indistinct, but the keratinized oral gingival epithelium is clearly seen with its regular deep rete pegs.
Fig. 2.8(b) shows the most apical portion of the junctional epithelium and corresponds to the diagram in Fig. 2.6. It should be noted that the junctional epithelium extends on to the acellular cementum covering the root surface for a short distance. The enamel space can be seen in the top left of the picture – it is important to note that this is not the gingival crevice.

healthy tissue (Fig. 2.7). These cells do not remain in the junctional epithelium, but pass through into the gingival crevice, where they play a crucial role in the host defence against micro-organisms in dental plaque.

Junctional epithelium turns over rapidly. Estimates of the length of time this tissue takes to renew itself range from 4–11 days, compared with about a month in other parts of the oral mucosa (see p. 26). Cell division takes place throughout the length of the junctional epithelium, with the cells being shed into the gingival sulcus. Under normal conditions the rate of production of new cells is balanced by the rate of desquamation into the sulcus. The regulation of turnover in junctional epithelium in health is discussed on pp. 25–6 and the changes which occur in periodontal disease are described in Chapter 3.

Junctional epithelium is highly adapted to its role of ensuring a firm and effective attachment between oral mucosa and the tooth surface. The level of differentiation which is necessary to permit the ready formation of hemidesmosomes along the enamel surface, as well as at the interface with connective tissue, is that usually found in cells of the basal layers. Thus, the cells within the junctional epithelium appear to be maintained at a fairly early stage of maturation and do not differentiate to the stage where membrane coating granule formation occurs. As a consequence of their absence, and because of the large intercellular spaces that are present, junctional epithelium is readily permeable to substances (notably some components of dental plaque) which may be present in the gingival crevice. The absence of a permeability barrier is important in facilitating the host response to the micro-organisms which accumulate in dental plaque at the gingival margin. However, it should be emphasized that the principal function of junctional epithelium is to maintain attachment of junctional epithelium to the tooth surface, and its structure is the result of its specialization for that function.

Junctional epithelium is formed when the reduced enamel epithelium fuses with the oral epithelium as the tooth erupts. As the tooth moves into occlusion, the attachment moves apically down the crown, stabilizing in the region of the amelo-cemental junction. It is important to note that the junctional epithelium re-forms on the root surface following periodontal surgery. Although this new junctional epithelium is derived entirely from oral epithelium, its structure is identical to normal junctional epithelium. This suggests that it is the relationship of the epithelium to the tooth surface and the underlying connective tissue, not its developmental origin, which is critical in determining the structure of junctional epithelium.

2.2.4 Gingival connective tissue

The principal components of the gingival connective tissues are collagen fibres, which account for approximately 60 per cent of its volume, and the extracellular matrix in which they are embedded. Together, these give the gingiva its strength and resilience. Fibroblasts synthesize both collagen and the extracellular matrix, and they are the predominant cell type. However, a small number of inflammatory cells, mostly macrophages and neutrophil polymorphonuclear leucocytes, may also be present. Lymphocytes may occasionally be seen around blood vessels deep within the connective tissue, forming the normal resident lymphocyte population. The gingiva is highly vascular, the blood vessels not only providing oxygen and nutrients for the maintenance of the connective tissue and overlying epithelia, but also a route of entry for circulating inflammatory cells when needed.

Most of the collagen fibres in the gingiva are arranged in groups with a distinctive orientation (Fig. 2.9) and together form a fibrous cuff around the tooth. The fibre groups include:

1. Circular fibres, present in the free gingiva and encircling the tooth.

2. Trans-septal fibres, which are attached into the most coronal portion of the cementum of adjacent teeth and run between them above the level of the inter-dental septum of the alveolar bone, so that they join the teeth together.

3. Dento-gingival fibres arise in the cementum above the level of the alveolar crest and fan out into the free gingiva.

4. Dento-periosteal fibres also arise in the cementum in the same region as the dento-gingival fibres and are distributed apically over the top of the alveolar crest, ending in the attached gingiva.

5. Crestal fibres, which run from the alveolar crest into the attached gingiva.

Collagen is synthesized by fibroblasts and secreted in an inactive form, procollagen, which is converted to tropocollagen. This is polymerized into collagen fibrils, which are then aggregated into collagen bundles by the formation of cross linkages. Different types of collagen exist and these exhibit variation in the composition of the basic tropocollagen molecule. The most common form found in gingiva is type I collagen, although type III and type V collagen are also present. The distribution of these collagen types differs within the gingiva, with type I collagen predominating in the deeper connective tissue and the finer type III collagen being found more superficially. Type V collagen accounts for only about 5 per cent of the total. In addition, type IV collagen is present in the basement membranes of capillaries and the overlying epithelium.

Fibroblasts secrete the other components of the extracellular matrix, in

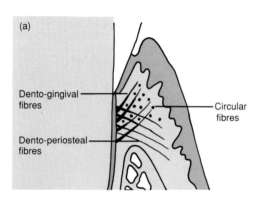

Fig. 2.9   The fibre types present in the gingiva, which together form a firm fibrous cuff around the neck of the tooth.
Fig. 2.9(a) shows the fibres seen on the buccal aspect (lingual and palatal aspects are essentially similar).

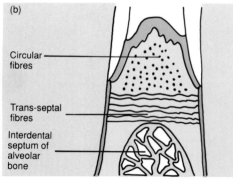

Fig. 2.9(b) shows the gingival fibres in the interdental area. Trans-septal fibres are seen in addition to those in Fig. 2.9(a).

addition to collagen fibres. These include the glycosaminoglycans (GAGs), proteoglycans, and glycoproteins. The most common GAG is hyaluronic acid, large amounts of which are found in gingiva. GAGs are linked to protein to form the much larger proteoglycans. These include heparin sulphate and dermatan sulphate which are present in gingiva. GAGs are long unbranched polysaccharides which have the property of binding large amounts of water. As a result, tissues containing significant amounts of GAG resist compressive forces and the transport of nutrients through the extracellular spaces is facilitated.

Although collagen is the most common protein found within gingiva, many others are also present. One of these is fibronectin, which is a large glycoprotein with the property of binding to cells, as well as to collagen and proteoglycans. It is important in promoting the adhesion of fibroblasts to the extracellular matrix and it also plays a role in the alignment of collagen fibres. The degradation of collagen and the other connective matrix components is discussed on pp. 26–8.

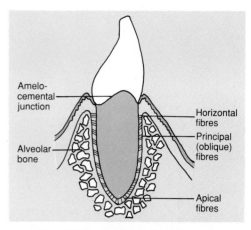

Fig. 2.10 Fibre types present in the periodontal ligament. The principal fibres make up the majority and accommodate the numerous small tooth movements associated with masticatory function. The horizontal fibres run between the alveolar crest and cementum. The apical fibres run radially between the tooth root and adjacent alveolar bone in the region of the tooth apex.

2.3 The periodontal ligament

The periodontal ligament is the fibrous attachment of the tooth inserting into cementum on the root and into the alveolar bone. The principal components of the ligament are the collagen fibres which, like the gingival fibres, are arranged in groups (Fig. 2.10).

The principal fibres run obliquely in an apical direction from the alveolar bone to the root of the tooth. These fibres have a somewhat wavy course, which accommodates the minor movements of the tooth in its socket during mastication and other functions in which tooth contact occurs. The ends of the principal fibres, which are embedded in alveolar bone and cementum, are referred to as Sharpey's fibres. These may mineralize around their periphery, but they usually retain an unmineralized core. The horizontal fibres run, as their name indicates, horizontally between the alveolar crest and the cementum covering the tooth root. The apical fibres run radially between alveolar bone and tooth in the region of the tooth apex.

As in gingiva, the main collagen types present within the periodontal ligament are types I, III, and V, with small amounts of type IV collagen in the basement membranes of blood vessels. Type III collagen is more fibrillar and extensible than type I and it is present in similar proportions to those found in embryonic and granulation tissue, which is probably a reflection of the high rate of collagen turnover within the periodontal ligament. The presence of the type III collagen may be important in maintaining the integrity of the ligament during the small vertical and horizontal tooth movements which occur during chewing.

Oxytalan fibres are also found in the periodontal ligament, but have not been found elsewhere in the body. These are elastic fibres which insert into cementum but run a more longitudinal course than other fibres. Although their function is unclear, they are more often seen in teeth bearing abnormal loads and may be associated with preservation of the position of blood vessels during occlusal loading.

The extracellular matrix of the periodontal ligament is similar to that of gingiva. Hyaluronic acid, heparin sulphate, chondroitin-4- and -6-sulphates, and dermatan sulphate are all present. These molecules, which turn over at an even faster rate than collagen, are important in binding water. They may thus act as a hydraulic cushion in the periodontal ligament, and this cushioning effect may be as important as traction on the periodontal fibres in withstanding the forces of mastication.

Fibroblasts are the main cell type present in the periodontal ligament. Because of the high turnover rate of the ligament, these cells are actively engaged in protein synthesis and appear plump with abundant cytoplasm. They are also responsible for the degradation of collagen in the periodontal ligament. The periodontal ligament has a rich nerve supply, is vascular, and contains cells which give rise to cementum and bone. These cells are important in the maintenance and repair of the periodontal ligament and its insertions into bone and cementum.

Cementoblasts line the surface of cementum and osteoblasts line the endosteal and periosteal surfaces of alveolar bone. Both of these cell types are only conspicuous when active deposition of cementum or bone is occurring, when they assume a plumper morphology. When either of these tissues is stimulated to resorb (see Chapter 3), multi-nucleate osteoclasts appear on their surfaces. The cells which resorb cementum are sometimes referred to as cementoclasts, but they appear identical to osteoclasts and, as osteoclasts have been shown capable of resorbing all biological mineralized substrates *in vitro*, there seems no reason to differentiate between them. The precursors of both the osteoblasts and cementoblasts which line the periodontal ligament are probably adjacent undifferentiated connective tissue cells, but osteoclasts are derived from blood-borne precursors which originate in the bone marrow. The periodontal ligament has a nerve supply, one of the important functions of which is the monitoring of loading during mastication. Proprioceptive fibres within the ligament are also involved in reflex salivation during chewing.

The other principal cells present within the periodontal ligament are the odontogenic epithelial cells which comprise the cell rests of Malassez. These cells, which are the remnants of Hertwig's root sheath, appear as isolated groups of darkly staining cells in routine light microscopy, but in reality they form a plexus which surrounds the tooth. Their function – if any – is unknown, but they may be involved in maintaining the integrity of the periodontal ligament and preventing ankylosis.

2.4 Alveolar bone

Alveolar bone is that part of the mandible and maxilla which surrounds and supports the roots of the teeth. It is 'tooth dependent' in that it develops in association with the teeth and is gradually resorbed if the teeth are lost. No distinct boundary exists to distinguish alveolar bone from that of the body of the mandible or maxilla. It is made up of cancellous (medullary) bone covered by a thin layer of compact (cortical) bone. The fibres of the periodontal ligament insert into the alveolar bone. It surrounds the roots of erupted teeth to within 1–2 mm of the amelo-cemental junction. Because of the difference in the level of this junction on mesial and distal tooth surfaces compared with its position on buccal (or labial) and lingual (or palatal) surfaces, the crest of the interproximal bone is usually more coronally positioned than that of the adjacent alveolar bone.

In common with the rest of the skeleton, alveolar bone is constantly turning over under the influence of systemic and locally produced factors which control bone homeostasis, and it can re-model in response to functional demands. The target cells for those factors stimulating resorption are osteoblasts, which line the periosteal and endosteal surfaces of alveolar bone as well as the lamina dura of the tooth sockets. These cells in turn instruct osteoclasts to remove bone, producing the typical Howship's lacunae seen in histological preparations of bone undergoing resorption. The turnover of alveolar bone and the regulation of this process is described on pp. 28–9.

2.5 Cementum

The cementum is important because it provides the site of anchorage of the periodontal ligament fibres on the tooth. It is a mineralized tissue, covering the entire root surface of the tooth and firmly bound to the underlying dentine. Cementum is similar in composition to bone, although it is avascular and not innervated. It occurs in two forms: acellular, which covers the entire root surface, and cellular, found near the apex of the tooth. At the amelo-cemental junction the cementum either abuts or slightly overlaps the enamel, except for a small minority of teeth where the cementum and enamel do not meet and dentine is exposed. The thickness of cementum increases throughout life and varies from 10 μm cervically to over 600 μm apically. One important difference in the behaviour of cementum and bone is that cementum is much less readily resorbed than bone, although the reasons for this are unclear.

2.6 Regulation of tissue turnover in the periodontium

The dynamic nature of the periodontium has already been emphasized. In health, the synthesis and breakdown of its components are carefully controlled and in balance, so that the tissues maintain their composition, volume, and integrity and are able to respond to functional demands. This concept is referred to as tissue homeostasis, and its regulation is generally under both local and systemic control.

Even in health, the rates of synthesis or tissue breakdown may alter, depending on functional demands. For instance, in the face of increased demand, the rate of synthesis of a tissue component may exceed its breakdown, resulting in a net accumulation. Conversely, if functional demands are decreased, breakdown may exceed synthesis, resulting in the net loss of that component. In either situation, a steady state will be reached once the tissue has adapted to the new functional demands. This concept of the regulation of turnover and maintenance of tissue integrity is important in understanding the changes that occur in periodontal disease. If the stresses on a tissue exceed its ability to adapt and respond then damage will occur. Thus the tissue destruction which occurs in periodontal disease may result from the perturbation of normal regulatory processes, exceeding the capacity of specific tissue components to respond within their normal adaptive range. It is possible that the periods when the homeostatic balance in a tissue is lost may be very short-lived and they probably correspond to the bursts of tissue destruction which were described in Chapter 1.

The mechanisms governing normal tissue turnover in the periodontium are discussed in this section and the factors which may upset homeostasis in disease will be dealt with in Chapter 6.

2.6.1 Epithelium

The keratinocytes in oral epithelium (see pp. 19–21) are continually shed from the surface, and in health these are replaced by an equal number of successors arising from cell division in the basal cell layers. Although most of the cells in the basal layers are capable of division, only a few retain the capacity to divide through life. These are known as stem cells and they are essential for renewal of the epithelium. The remainder have a limited capacity for division before they start to differentiate and move up into the prickle cell or spinous layer (see Fig. 2.4). The time taken for the cells within the epithelium to be shed and completely replaced by new cells is defined as the 'turnover time' for that epithelium. This varies greatly between different sites; the turnover time for skin is 12–75 days and for oral gingival epithelium it varies between 8 and 40 days. Junctional epithelium has one of the fastest epithelial turnover times in the body at between 4 and 11 days.

Epithelial turnover is influenced by factors which affect the rate of cell division, the maturation and movement of cells through the prickle cell layers, and the rate of desquamation. Systemic hormones affect cell division within epithelium; oestrogens stimulate the process whereas adrenaline and corticosteroids have the opposite effect. However, local factors play a more important role in regulating cell division than these hormones.

Early studies on epithelial cell division suggested the existence of a negative feedback control system by which keratinocytes in the prickle cell layer produced substances called chalones which acted on the proliferating cells in the basal layers to inhibit their division. The precise nature of these chalones is not known and it is likely that their action will eventually be attributed to cytokines. These are proteins or glycoproteins which are produced by a variety of cell types and which regulate the growth and differentiation of other cells. Cytokines usually act locally, although some have a systemic action. Epithelial turnover appears to be affected by at least three cytokines: epidermal growth factor (EGF), transforming growth factor alpha (TFGα), and transforming growth factor beta (TGFβ). Although the exact role these cytokines play in the regulation of cell division in normal epithelium is uncertain, TGFα and EGF can stimulate proliferation and it is probable that TGFβ has an inhibitory effect, as well as promoting differentiation (see Table 2.1).

In addition to the action of cytokines such as TGFβ, the pattern of epithelial differentiation is influenced by the underlying connective tissue. For example, the differentiation of the junctional epithelium is probably determined, at least in part, by the adjacent connective tissue of the periodontal ligament (see p. 21). The extent to which the pattern of epithelial differentiation seen at different sites is due to stable intrinsic difference in the keratinocytes is not known. The homeostatic mechanisms described in this section may be perturbed in periodontal disease, perhaps due to the increased production of cytokines accompanying the inflammatory response. These events are discussed further in Chapters 5 and 6.

Table 2.1 Cytokines which influence keratinocyte division

Stimulate	Inhibit
TGFα	TGFβ
EGF	

2.6.2 Connective tissue

In health, the gingival connective tissues (see pp. 22–3) undergo continual turnover, with the rates of synthesis and degradation in a state of equilibrium. Connective tissue turnover varies widely between tissues and it is particularly rapid in the periodontal ligament. Turnover here is five times higher than in alveolar bone and fifteen times greater than in normal skin.

Fibroblasts are responsible for both synthesis and degradation of extracellular matrix. The synthesis of collagen and the other matrix components was described on pp. 22–3. Enzymes capable of degrading collagen are also secreted by fibroblasts. These collagenases form part of a group of enzymes known as metalloproteinases because they require the presence of such divalent cations as calcium and magnesium for their activity. Other enzymes in this group include proteoglycanase, or stromelysin, and gelatinase which degrade proteoglycans and other matrix components. Collagenases cleave small segments of collagen fibrils from larger collagen fibre bundles at a site specific to the collagen type. These segments are taken up by fibroblasts and digested intracellularly by their lysosomal enzymes (Fig. 2.11). Collagenases are powerful enzymes with the potential to cause marked connective tissue destruction. To control their activity and prevent unwanted tissue damage, a number of important mechanisms exist. Collagenases are secreted in an inactive form bound to collagen. In normal healthy tissues their activity is low, although little is known about the factors controlling their activation. However, there is some evidence that tissue proteinases, such as plasminogen activating factor, may be important. The most important regulators of metalloproteinase activity appear to be tissue inhibitors of metalloproteinases (TIMP). These, as well as collagenases, are secreted by fibroblasts, and are thought to be an important safeguard against excessive matrix degradation. Failure of TIMP to suppress the activity of metalloproteinases can lead to significant tissue injury.

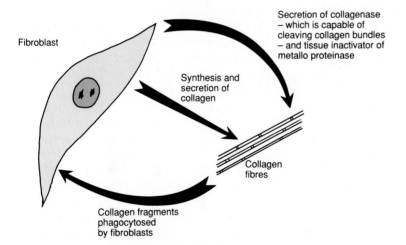

Fibroblast

Secretion of collagenase – which is capable of cleaving collagen bundles – and tissue inactivator of metallo proteinase

Synthesis and secretion of collagen

Collagen fibres

Collagen fragments phagocytosed by fibroblasts

Fig. 2.11 The processes involved in collagen homeostasis. Fibroblasts synthesize and secrete collagen. They also secrete collagenase, a metalloproteinase in a latent form, and TIMP. On being activated, metalloproteinases cleave the collagen fibres into small fragments, which are subsequently phagocytosed by the fibroblast. Excessive or inappropriate metalloproteinase activation is normally prevented by TIMP.

Little is known about how connective tissue turnover is regulated. Systemic factors are probably of major importance during growth and development, but the extent to which they play an important regulatory role in health at other times is uncertain. Very little is known about the role of cytokines and other local factors in connective tissue turnover in health; several have been shown to stimulate production by fibroblasts of collagen, fibronectin, and gly-cosaminogycans *in vitro*. These include platelet derived growth factor (PDGF), fibroblast growth factors (FGF), and TGFβ. On the other hand, cytokines such as interleukin 1 (Il-1) and interferon gamma (IFNγ) have been shown to stimulate the production of collagenase (Table 2.2). However, before a role in normal turnover can be assigned to these cytokines more research is required to establish whether they are present in health, and if they are active at physiological concentrations.

Table 2.2 Cytokines which influence turnover of connective tissues

Stimulate secretion of collagen and GAGs	Stimulate secretion of collagenase
PDGF	IFNγ
FGF	Il-1
TGFβ	

2.6.3 Bone

Bone turns over continually throughout life, with bone deposition mediated by osteoblasts linked or 'coupled' with resorption mediated by osteoclasts, so that the volume of bone remains relatively constant in health. This re-modelling serves two important functions: the maintenance of blood calcium levels within the normal range and adaptation to changes in mechanical loading. Osteoblasts are responsible for both the synthesis and calcification of the bone matrix. Initially, an uncalcified matrix or osteoid is formed, and this subsequently mineralizes as a result of the deposition of crystals of hydroxyapatite. These are initially associated with structures called matrix vesicles, derived from the cytoplasm of osteoblasts, but as the process progresses mineralization also involves the collagen fibres (Fig. 2.12).

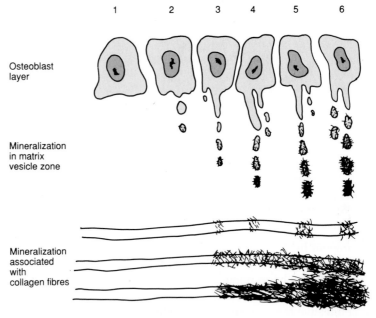

Fig. 2.12 The events occurring during early mineralization. The osteoblasts secrete bone matrix as unmineralized osteoid (1) and then extrude matrix vesicles into the osteoid zone (2). These structures are able to concentrate calcium, and initial mineralization occurs within the matrix vesicles (2–3). As these events progress, the underlying structure of the matrix vesicles becomes obscured (5) and mineral crystals begin to deposit on the collagen fibres embedded in the matrix. This process appears initially to correspond to the banding of collagen fibres (3–4), but as it progresses the entire fibre becomes involved. Subsequently (5–6), mineralization begins to involve the interfibrillar matrix, so that the collagen fibres are no longer visible (6). This sequence is hypothetical at present, and the link between initial mineralization in matrix vesicles and subsequent mineralization of collagen fibres and the interfibrillar matrix is not known.

Osteoclasts are only evident at sites undergoing resorption, when they are found closely applied to the bone surface in pits or depressions known as Howship's lacunae. Numerous vesicles are evident within the cytoplasm of active osteoclasts, and these contain a wide range of hydrolytic enzymes important in bone resorption. Initially, osteoclasts de-mineralize the bone matrix and then degrade the residual collagen.

Little is known about the mechanism which links bone resorption to deposition, but bone matrix contains numerous growth factors which may be released during resorption and these might stimulate the differentiation of osteoblasts and the deposition of bone. Although bone resorption is mediated by osteoclasts, many of the agents which stimulate resorption, such as parathyroid hormone (PTH), act on the osteoblast and not on the osteoclast itself (Fig. 2.13). Osteoblasts respond to PTH by releasing osteoclast stimulating factor, which probably acts directly on the osteoclast to stimulate resorption. Osteoblasts also release collagenase, which may be important in removing the superficial layer of unmineralized osteoid present on the bone surface. As a result, hydroxyapatite crystals are exposed, and it is thought that this is critical in initiating osteoclastic bone resorption.

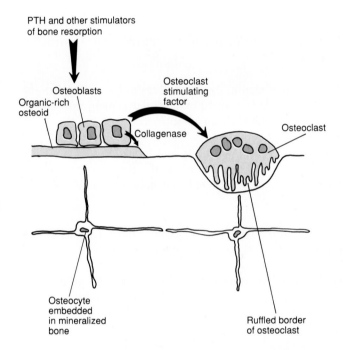

Fig. 2.13 How the interaction of bone resorbing agents with osteoblasts leads to increased osteoclastic activity. Collagenase produced by osteoblasts degrades the superficial organic matrix, exposing bone mineral to osteoclast attack. In addition, osteoclasts are activated by osteoclast stimulating factor secreted by osteoblasts. The osteoclast cell membrane in contact with the bone is deeply infolded, or 'ruffled', increasing its surface area. The cell synthesizes hydrolytic enzymes in vesicles which fuse with the ruffled border and are released into the space between the osteoclast, leading to degradation of bone mineral and the matrix.

In addition to the systemically acting factors involved in bone homeostasis, such as PTH and calcitonin, a number of substances have been identified which are capable of stimulating bone resorption *in vitro* and which could be involved in the local control of bone turnover. These agents include prostaglandin E2 (PGE2) and cytokines such as Il-1, and tumour necrosis factors alpha (TNFα) and beta (TNFβ). The significance that these factors have in normal bone homeostasis is unknown, but they are generated in the course of inflammatory and immune responses and may play a role in periodontal disease, as discussed in Chapters 5 and 6.

2.7 Summary

1. The periodontium attaches the teeth to the jaws and supports them during masticatory function. Principal components are the gingiva, periodontal ligament, alveolar bone, and cementum.

2. The gingiva is composed of epithelium and connective tissue. The keratinized oral gingival epithelium protects the underlying connective tissue during mastication. The junctional epithelium attaches the epithelium lining the mouth to the teeth.

3. Gingival connective tissues are composed of collagen fibres embedded in an extracellular matrix. The collagen fibres are arranged into circular fibres, trans-septal fibres, dento-gingival fibres, and dento-periosteal fibres.

4. The main components of the periodontal ligament are the principal, horizontal, and apical fibres. Sharpey's fibres are the portions of the principal fibres inserted into bone and cementum. The extracellular matrix contains hyaluronic acid, heparin sulphate, chondroitin sulphate, and dermatan sulphate.

5. Alveolar bone is that part of the mandible and maxilla which surrounds and supports the teeth.

6. Cementum anchors the periodontal ligament fibres to the surfaces of the tooth. The entire root surface is covered by acellular cementum; cellular cementum may be present near the root apex.

7. Homeostatic mechanisms control synthesis and breakdown of the components of the periodontium in health, enable the tissues to respond to functional demands, and maintain a balance between these opposing effects.

8. Junctional epithelium and the periodontal ligament have a relatively fast turnover. This is regulated by cytokines and other local factors.

9. Collagen turnover is under the control of fibroblasts. In addition to secreting collagen and matrix components, they also produce metalloproteinases, responsible for enzymatic breakdown of the tissue, and tissue inactivators of metalloproteinases (TIMP).

10. Bone turnover results from the interaction of osteoblasts and osteoclasts. Local factors regulating their activity include cytokines and prostaglandins.

2.8 Further reading

Berkowitz, B.M.B., Moxham, B.J., and Newman, H.N. (1982). *Periodontal ligament in health and disease*. (Pergamon, Oxford).
— *A useful general reference.*

Gage, J.P., Francis, M.J.O., and Triffitt, J.T. (1990). *Collagen and dental matrices*. (Wright, London).
— *An excellent account of the connective tissue matrix.*

Marks, S.C. and Popoff, S.N. (1988). Bone cell biology: the regulation of development, structure and function in the skeleton. *Amer. J. Anat.* **183**, 1–44.
— *An excellent, up-to-date review of the key aspects of bone structure, function, and turnover.*

Schroeder, H.E. and Listgarten, M.A. (1971). *Fine structure of the developing attachment of human teeth*. (Karger, Basel).
— *Although published 20 years ago, this is a milestone work on the structure of the periodontium.*

Squier, C.A., Johnson, N.W., and Hopps, R.M. (1976). *Human oral mucosa*. (Blackwell, Oxford).
— *A good basic account of oral mucosa.*

Ten Cate, A.R. (1989). *Oral histology: development, structure and function*, 3rd edn. (Mosby, St Louis).
— *Good basic accounts of the structure of the periodontium and oral mucosa.*

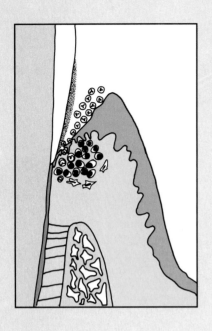

3 The anatomy of periodontal disease

3.1 Introduction

This chapter describes the sequence of events occurring in the initially healthy periodontium in response to the accumulation of dental plaque. It was pointed out in Chapter 1 that the nature of the host response, as well as differences in the microbial flora, will give rise to recognizably different clinical forms of periodontal disease. However, these do not appear to differ significantly in their histological appearance. The changes described in this chapter assume a relentless progression from initial gingivitis to advanced periodontal disease, with marked bone loss leading eventually to exfoliation of teeth. However, this is a somewhat artificial view, because in most cases the disease remains at the stage of established, but stable, gingivitis. Progression, when it occurs, is usually both localized and episodic.

Knowledge of the pathological events occurring during the course of periodontal disease is based heavily on experimental studies, using either human subjects or experimental animals. In the majority of these, plaque is allowed to accumulate once the gingivae have been rendered healthy by professional tooth cleaning. It should, therefore, be realized that the time-scale of the events described here is probably different from that in naturally occurring disease. The factors which affect disease progression include changes in the microbial flora, discussed in Chapter 4, and host factors, described in Chapter 5. Nevertheless, the stages in the disease process described in this chapter serve as a framework for the discussion of the pathogenic mechanisms in subsequent chapters.

The changes which occur in the periodontium constitute a continuum, but, for the purpose of relating them to the clinical stages of disease, they will be described under the headings of:

(1) early gingivitis – includes the stages sometimes referred to as the 'initial lesion' and the 'early lesion';

(2) chronic marginal gingivitis – sometimes referred to as the 'established lesion';

(3) destructive periodontitis – sometimes referred to as the 'advanced lesion'.

3.2 Early gingivitis

3.2.1 The first week (the initial lesion)

Clinical changes take between one or two weeks to appear after the initial accumulation of supragingival dental plaque at the gingival margin, and do not become marked until three or more weeks. By this stage, the gingivae will have become somewhat swollen and reddened, exhibiting a tendency to bleed readily on gentle probing. However, more subtle changes are apparent during the first week of plaque accumulation, and these are associated with the fluid phase of acute inflammation. Crevicular fluid flow increases within the first 24 hours, as a result of the increased permeability of the blood vessels adjacent to the junctional epithelium. Crevicular fluid is essentially an inflammatory exudate and contains the typical constituents, such as plasma proteins, immuno-globulins, and complement components. However, it is modified during its passage through the crevice by the addition of bacterial products and components derived from connective tissue breakdown. The increase in crevicular fluid flow begins during the first week, but does not become marked until about

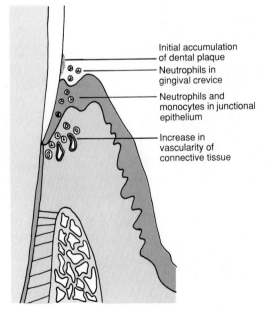

Initial accumulation of dental plaque

Neutrophils in gingival crevice

Neutrophils and monocytes in junctional epithelium

Increase in vascularity of connective tissue

Fig. 3.1 Early gingivitis – the first week.

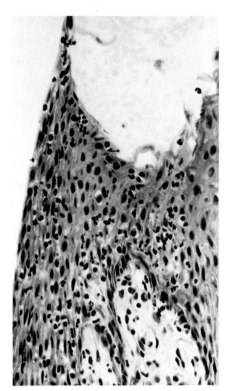

Fig. 3.2 Photomicrograph of the coronal part of the junctional epithelium and the base of the gingival crevice. This is in the top right of the figure. The enamel space is present in the top left corner.

Numerous neutrophils, with their small darkly-staining nuclei, can be seen in the junctional epithelium, passing between the epithelial cells as they migrate into the gingival crevice.

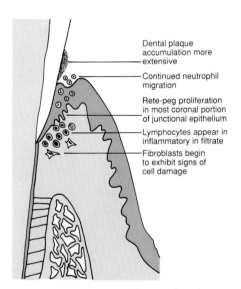

Dental plaque accumulation more extensive

Continued neutrophil migration

Rete-peg proliferation in most coronal portion of junctional epithelium

Lymphocytes appear in inflammatory in filtrate

Fibroblasts begin to exhibit signs of cell damage

Fig. 3.3 Early gingivitis – the second week.

10 days after the initial accumulation of dental plaque. It is accompanied by an increase in the vascularity of the underlying connective tissue as a result of dilatation of blood vessels and, probably, endothelial cell proliferation (Fig. 3.1).

The vascular events of the acute inflammatory response are also accompanied by cellular events. Although small numbers of neutrophils are present in junctional epithelium in health (Fig. 2.7), their numbers increase sharply following plaque accumulation (Fig. 3.2). Large numbers of neutrophils are also seen in the gingival crevice and, to a lesser extent, in the adjacent connective tissue. This begins at around 24 hours and becomes marked and persistent after 4–5 days. Smaller numbers of monocytes and macrophages are also found in the junctional epithelium, crevice and connective tissue.

Although the cell infiltrate shows the features of an acute inflammatory reaction at this early stage, small numbers of lymphocytes may be seen during the first week. These cells become far more conspicuous as the inflammatory infiltrate becomes established. Within the area of the inflammatory infiltrate there is a marked loss of perivascular collagen, with a reduction of up to 70 per cent of the amount normally found in uninflamed areas.

3.2.2 The second week (the early lesion)

As the growth of supragingival plaque continues and becomes more extensive, the features described above become more marked and the inflammatory infiltrate enlarges to occupy a greater volume of the gingiva (Fig. 3.3). This is accompanied by a shift in the cell population, with an increase in the number of lymphocytes and macrophages. The lymphocytes appear as small round cells, with darkly staining nuclei and an inconspicuous rim of cytoplasm. Both T and B cells are present, and these increase in number, with T cells dominating the infiltrate towards the end of this stage.

Two other features become evident during the second week of plaque accumulation. Fibroblasts begin to show signs of cell damage, and there is marked collagen loss near the junctional epithelium. A hyperplastic response is also seen at the most coronal part of the junctional epithelium itself, with rete-peg proliferation (Figs 3.3 and 3.4).

It should be realized that, although the features of chronic inflammation come to dominate the lesion as time progresses, the features of acute inflammation persist, with marked crevicular fluid flow and continued neutrophil emigration into the gingival crevice.

3.3 Chronic marginal gingivitis (the established lesion)

In areas where plaque accumulation has been allowed to persist for two to three weeks the clinical features of chronic marginal gingivitis are seen (Fig. 3.5). The gingival margins and interdental papillae are more markedly reddened and oedematous than in the initial stages of gingivitis. Crevicular fluid flow may be evident clinically and the gingivae bleed readily on gentle probing. This situation can remain stable for long periods of time. In many individuals it may never progress, and it heals readily with improved oral hygiene.

The inflammatory infiltrate in the connective tissue is increased substantially in volume, extending apically and laterally (Fig. 3.6), although it is still in contact with the junctional epithelium. Perivascular accumulation of chronic inflammatory cells is also evident at this stage, possibly reflecting a higher rate of inflammatory cell emigration. Although macrophages are present throughout the infiltrate in the established lesion of chronic marginal gingivitis, lymphocytes are the dominant cell type. Many of the B cells will have matured into plasma cells, and these account for the majority of the population. They are actively engaged in the synthesis of immunoglobulin, which is released locally into the surrounding connective tissue. This immunoglobulin passes through the junctional epithelium, to enter the gingival crevice as one of the important components of crevicular fluid.

The lateral proliferation of junctional epithelium, first noticed in early gingivitis (Fig. 3.4), becomes marked in chronic marginal gingivitis. This affects the coronal portion of junctional epithelium, but there is no significant apical migration of the epithelial attachment (Fig. 3.6). The epithelium becomes thinned and detached from the tooth surface in places and ulceration may be seen. Largely as a result of gingival swelling, the gingival crevice becomes deepened, although true pocket formation does not occur because there is no loss of connective tissue attachment. In the deepened gingival crevice anaerobic conditions begin to develop and, as the dental plaque extends downward, there is a substantial shift in the flora as it adapts to the more anaerobic conditions which prevail in the deepest parts. Thus the microbial flora of subgingival plaque differs significantly from supragingival plaque. This is discussed in more detail in Chapter 4.

The emigration of neutrophils into the gingival crevice becomes more marked in chronic marginal gingivitis and these cells attach themselves to the surface of the subgingival plaque, forming a barrier between it and the junctional epithelium. The epithelium itself is also more heavily infiltrated by inflammatory cells than previously as a consequence of their increased migration into the gingival crevice.

The increase in the extent of the chronic inflammatory infiltrate is accompanied by marked collagen loss in the involved connective tissue, but no loss of alveolar bone or connective tissue attachment is seen in chronic marginal gingivitis.

Many complex interrelated events occur in the tissues in chronic marginal gingivitis, as discussed in Chapters 5 and 6, but this condition represents the stable interaction between the micro-organisms in dental plaque and host defence reactions. Consequently, although there is substantial cell emigration

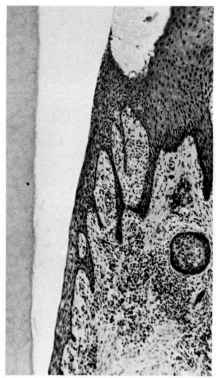

Fig. 3.4 Early gingivitis – the second week. Junctional epithelium shows rete-peg proliferation in the coronal portion. The enamel space (which resulted from de-mineralisation of the specimen during preparation) can be seen adjacent to the junctional epithelium on the left side. In the connective tissue beneath the epithelium on the right side the inflammatory infiltrate can be seen. Compare these appearances with the features shown diagrammatically in Fig. 3.3.

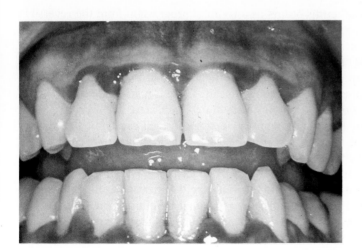

Fig. 3.5 Chronic marginal gingivitis involving the attached gingiva around the upper incisors. There is marked oedema and reddening in response to plaque accumulation. This is especially marked in the interdental papillae between the upper right central and lateral incisor teeth.

and increased tissue turnover in the periodontium, there may be no progression in attachment loss over a long period of time. Destructive periodontal disease will only occur when there is an imbalance in these interactions in favour of tissue breakdown, due either to changes in the host defence mechanisms or the plaque flora. The mechanisms thought to lead to destruction are evaluated in Chapter 6.

3.4 Destructive periodontitis (the advanced lesion)

Destructive periodontitis may present in a number of clinically distinct forms, as discussed in Chapter 1. The typical appearance of adult periodontitis is seen in Fig. 3.7, with loss of connective tissue attachment and fibrosis. Although marked alveolar bone loss is detectable radiographically at this stage (Fig. 3.8), there may be little evidence of gingival recession (Fig. 3.9). The more advanced features are illustrated in Fig. 3.10. There may now be marked apical migration of the gingival crest, reflecting the loss of underlying bone, and extensive supragingival plaque accumulation. A common observation, even at this advanced stage, is that the periodontium is not uniformly affected and some areas may remain relatively normal.

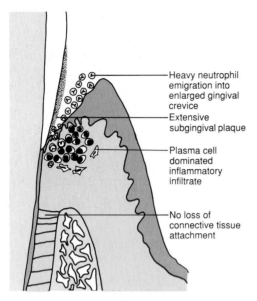

Fig. 3.6   Chronic marginal gingivitis.

Heavy neutrophil emigration into enlarged gingival crevice
Extensive subgingival plaque
Plasma cell dominated inflammatory infiltrate
No loss of connective tissue attachment

Fig. 3.7   Clinical appearance of adult periodontitis. The attached gingivae are grossly swollen, as a result of both oedema and fibrosis. There is gingival recession, especially interdentally, which is indicative of connective tissue attachment loss. This is particularly noticeable around the left lateral incisor tooth.

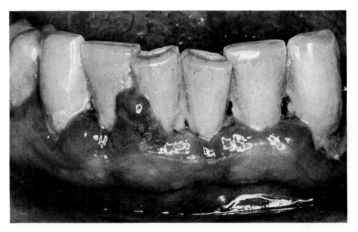

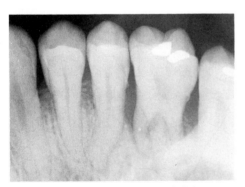

Fig. 3.8   Radiographic appearance of adult periodontitis affecting upper premolar and molar teeth. Although there is only slight loss of vertical bone height interproximally between the premolars, there has been severe bone loss around the first molar. This has almost reached the apices of the mesio-buccal and disto-buccal roots.

Destructive periodontitis occurs as a result of progression from the reversible damage seen in chronic marginal gingivitis to the irreversible destruction of periodontal support, with associated alveolar bone resorption (see Chapter 6). Many of the histological features described in chronic marginal gingivitis (Fig. 3.6) persist, and in a number of respects the inflammatory infiltrate is similar, although significant additional changes occur. There is marked apical migration and lateral extension of junctional epithelium, with areas of ulceration. This is associated with loss of the connective tissue attachment and the clinical consequence of this process is that true pocket formation is now seen. The loss of soft tissue apposition to the tooth surface which is part of this process permits extension of subgingival plaque on to the root surface.

The inflammatory infiltrate in the connective tissue becomes more extensive than in chronic marginal gingivitis, but it is similar in composition. At its deepest extent it is often focal and perivascular, with bands of fibrous tissue separating the foci. Collagen loss is directly associated with the inflammatory infiltrate, but fibrosis occurs at a distance. This gives rise to the irregular fibrotic appearance of the gingivae seen in advanced periodontal disease (Fig. 3.7).

Periodontal destruction is typically episodic, with bursts of destruction punctuated by periods of quiescence. Osteoclasts are not present in significant numbers on the surface of the alveolar bone adjacent to the inflammatory infiltrate during the quiescent phase, but during active resorption they may be present in large numbers (see Chapter 6). It appears likely that, even during periods of active osteoclast-mediated bone destruction, the inflammatory infiltrate does not impinge directly on the alveolar bone. This is a contentious point, however, because the methods presently available do not permit phases of active destruction to be identified with any certainty. However, in the numerous studies which have been undertaken, both in man and experimental animals, the inflammatory infiltrate is usually separated from the underlying bone by a zone of apparently normal connective tissue.

As with the established lesion of chronic marginal gingivitis, the advanced lesion may become stable. However, if progressive destruction occurs, bone loss may be so marked that the teeth become mobile and eventually exfoliate. A further complication of destructive periodontitis is that episodes of acute inflammation may occur, leading to the formation of periodontal abscesses. This may result in rapid and severe bone loss unless there is intervention to drain the abscess.

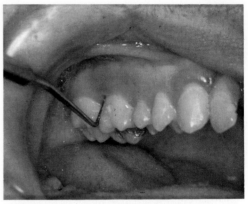

Fig. 3.9 Adult periodontitis affecting the upper molar teeth. Although there is little evidence of gingival recession, and the disease appears less severe than that in Fig. 3.7, there is significant loss of attachment between the first and second molar teeth. The periodontal probe has been inserted into a pocket which is 6mm deep on the distal aspect of the first molar.

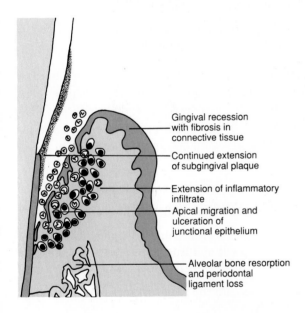

Gingival recession with fibrosis in connective tissue

Continued extension of subgingival plaque

Extension of inflammatory infiltrate

Apical migration and ulceration of junctional epithelium

Alveolar bone resorption and periodontal ligament loss

Fig. 3.10 Destructive periodontitis – the advanced lesion.

3.5 Summary

1. Although the clinical and histological changes which occur in the periodontium following plaque accumulation constitute a continuum, the following stages can be identified:

   (i) early gingivitis, includes the stages sometimes referred to as the 'initial lesion' and the 'early lesion';

   (ii) chronic marginal gingivitis, sometimes referred to as the 'established lesion';

  (iii) destructive periodontitis, sometimes referred to as the 'advanced lesion'.

2. Early gingivitis. Changes seen in the first week following the accumulation of dental plaque include:

  (i) swollen, reddened gingivae, which bleed readily on probing;

  (ii) increased crevicular fluid flow;

  (iii) histological features of acute inflammation with increased numbers of neutrophils in junctional epithelium and gingival crevice. Smaller numbers of monocytes, macrophages, and lymphocytes accumulate adjacent to the junctional epithelium. Vascularity increases and there is significant perivascular collagen loss within the area of the inflammatory infiltrate.

During the second week the features described above persist and the infiltrate becomes more extensive. In addition:

  (i) the connective tissue infiltrate becomes dominated by lymphocytes and macrophages;

  (ii) fibroblasts begin to show signs of cell damage, and there is marked collagen loss adjacent to the junctional epithelium;

  (iii) hyperplastic changes begin to appear in the most coronal part of the junctional epithelium, with proliferation of rete-pegs.

3. Chronic marginal gingivitis is characterized clinically by more marked oedema and reddening of the gingival margins and interdental papillae than in early gingivitis. This condition may remain stable for long periods of time and heals readily. In addition:

  (i) the volume of the inflammatory infiltrate is increased with apical and lateral extension;

  (ii) plasma cells predominate in the inflammatory infiltrate;

  (iii) rete-peg proliferation of junctional epithelium increases;

  (iv) the gingival crevice becomes deepened due to gingival swelling, but there is no loss of attachment and true pocket formation does not occur;

  (v) emigration of neutrophils into the gingival crevice becomes more marked than previously.

4. Destructive periodontitis occurs when interaction between micro-organisms in dental plaque and host defence reactions becomes unstable. It is characterized by true pocket formation and loss of alveolar bone, but destruction of bone occurs in bursts separated by periods of quiescence which may be lengthy. The histological features include:

  (i) marked apical migration and lateral extension of junctional epithelium, with areas of ulceration;

  (ii) loss of connective tissue attachment, resulting in true pocket formation;

(iii) extensive chronic inflammatory infiltrate in connective tissue adjacent to junctional epithelium. The composition of the infiltrate is essentially similar to that seen in chronic marginal gingivitis. At its deepest extent the infiltrate may be focal, with inflammatory cell accumulations separated by bands of fibrous tissue.

3.6 Further reading

Page, R.C. and Schroeder, H.E. (1976). Pathogenesis of inflammatory periodontal disease. A summary of current work. *Lab.Invest.* **33**, 235–49.

Page, R.C. and Schroeder, H.E. (1986). *Periodontitis in man and other animals.* (Karger, Basel).

Rateitschak, K.H., Rateitschak, E.M., Wolf, H.F., and Hassell, T.M. (1989). *Periodontology* 2nd edn. (Thieme, Stuttgart).

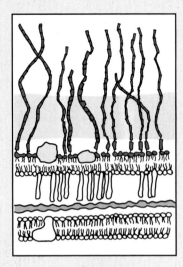

4 Microbial factors in the pathogenesis of periodontal disease

This chapter describes the role of plaque, its constituent micro-organisms, and their products in the pathogenesis of periodontal disease, starting with a definition of microbial plaque and a discussion of its variability and complexity. The subsequent section demonstrates why plaque is believed to be the prime aetiological agent in periodontal disease, using evidence from animal and human studies, including experimental gingivitis and microbiological studies. A detailed description of plaque is given on pp. 41–4. The accumulation of plaque with time and the formation of subgingival plaque and calculus is dealt with on pp. 44–8, while pp. 49–52 show how plaque differs under each of these conditions and emphasizes how the constant variation in plaque microbiology is a result of environmental pressures, such as competition for nutrients between species. The final section (pp. 52–64) describes how and why plaque may cause tissue damage, firstly by non-specific means, such as its physical nature and release of soluble factors, and secondly by the presence of specific microbial species within the plaque. A number of such potential pathogenic species are listed and their possible relationships to tissue damage discussed.

4.1 Microbial plaque and its significance

4.1.1 Microbial plaque

There is no doubt that dental or microbial plaque is the primary aetiological agent in periodontal disease, although the precise cause of the tissue damage which occurs remains unclear. Plaque comprises the bacterial aggregations adhering to teeth or oral mucosa; it is complex and in a continual state of change. Plaque consists of differing proportions of sticky matrix material and embedded bacteria. The matrix is derived partly from host products, such as salivary glycoprotein, dead cells, and serum proteins, and partly from bacterial products such as polysaccharides. The amount of matrix is variable; it accounts for about 50 per cent of supragingival plaque but there is almost none in deep

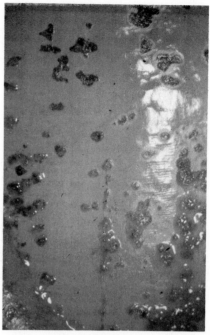

Fig. 4.1 Plaque colonies visible on anterior tooth a few days after ceasing toothbrushing. The colonies have been disclosed with a red vegetable dye to make them visible more readily. Separate colonies of 'pioneer' bacteria may be seen.

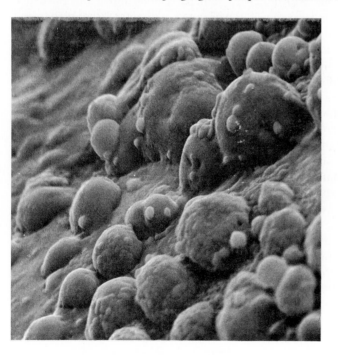

Fig. 4.2 Scanning electron micrograph showing early plaque, consisting of single and small colonies of coccal bacteria attached to the tooth surface by extracellular matrix.

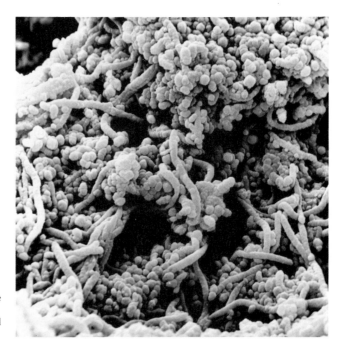

Fig. 4.3 Scanning electron micrograph showing the surface of mature supragingival plaque. There are filamentous bacteria at right angles to the surface and many cocci adhering to them.

subgingival plaque. The appearance of plaque on teeth is shown in Figs. 4.1–4.3.

4.1.2 Evidence for the role of plaque in periodontal disease

No single piece of evidence proves that plaque causes periodontal disease, but the weight of evidence overwhelmingly supports this view. There is excellent evidence to link plaque with gingivitis, but its relationship with destructive periodontal disease is more complex. It was noted in Chapter 1 that plaque and gingivitis are commonly found in the population, but that destructive periodontal disease is not. Thus the accumulation of plaque alone is most unlikely to be the sole cause of destructive periodontal disease, and other more specific changes may be responsible. Such changes could occur in the plaque flora, as discussed later in this chapter, or in the resistance of the host, as discussed in Chapter 5.

Cross-sectional epidemiological studies in man during the 1950s and 1960s showed that the degree of gingival inflammation and severity of periodontal disease correlated with the amount of dental plaque present in the mouth as a whole, and that localized areas of periodontal disease were associated with plaque 'traps' (calculus, faulty restorations and other so called 'secondary' or local factors). However, in 1965 a longitudinal study by Loe and co-workers established a model of experimental gingivitis and this has subsequently become a standard technique for investigating the initiation of gingivitis. A group of subjects with no gingival inflammation refrained from all oral hygiene measures for three weeks, during which time plaque deposits and gingival inflammation steadily increased. Reinstatement of oral hygiene measures subsequently resulted in plaque removal and a return to gingival health during the following week. Chlorhexidine mouthwashes have the same effect, confirming that it is the removal of plaque, rather than any mechanical effect, which is responsible for the return of gingival health.

Numerous clinical trials over the last 20 years or so have confirmed what dentists observe daily: that plaque control is effective in controlling gingivitis and periodontitis. Other forms of treatment aimed at killing or inhibiting bacteria have also been shown to be effective in reducing the extent and severity of periodontal disease. Such methods include the local application of the antiseptic agent chlorhexidine, which has been studied extensively, and the use of both topical and systemic antibiotics.

Animal studies have also been important in establishing the role of plaque in the aetiology of periodontal disease. The relationship between these animal models and human chronic periodontal disease is not immediately obvious, because the dental anatomy, oral flora, immune system, and rate and pattern of disease vary considerably from that found in humans. However, the results from animal studies generally correlate well with the evidence obtained under less well defined experimental circumstances in man, and some experiments, such as monoculture, are only possible in animals. The severity of periodontal disease in animals correlates with the general level of plaque accumulation and also to excessive local deposits. In ligature-induced periodontitis, for example, ligatures are tied around the cervical margin of a tooth in order to promote local plaque accumulation. Rapid periodontal breakdown results at the site but, in the absence of further manipulation, the disease often becomes stable after a period of destruction. Ligatures do not promote periodontal breakdown in germ-free animals, indicating that dental plaque is required for destruction and not just the ligature.

Some of the most convincing evidence that single strains of commensal oral bacteria are capable of causing periodontal disease comes from animal studies using the techniques of gnotobiosis and monoculture. These studies are performed using animals maintained in either germ-free or microbiologically controlled environments. Totally germ-free animals do not suffer the periodontal destruction seen under normal conditions, but when single strains of certain oral bacteria are introduced (monoculture experiments) rapid periodontal breakdown results. The destruction is often much more rapid and severe than in normal

Table 4.1 Evidence associating plaque with gingivitis and periodontal disease

Human studies
    Cross sectional and longitudinal epidemiological studies
    Experimental gingivitis
    Effectiveness of plaque control in the prevention of disease
    Effectiveness of plaque control in treatment of disease
    Effectiveness of chlorhexidine and antibiotics in treatment
    Reduced disease levels in patients on long term antimicrobial therapy

Animal studies
    Ligature induced periodontal disease
    Gnotobiotic and monoculture studies
    Experimental gingivitis in animals, especially dogs

Microbiological studies
    Correlation between disease and certain microbial species
    Potential virulence factors exist for some plaque bacteria

Immunological studies
    Association of antibody levels with specific bacteria

animals, possibly because gnotobiotic animals do not have a fully developed immune system. Such experiments have implicated many bacterial species in the causation of periodontal disease, including *Actinomyces viscosus* and *A. naeslundii*, *Actinobacillus actinomycetemcomitans*, *Porphyromonas gingivalis*, *Fusobacterium nucleatum*, *Capnocytophaga* sp., *Eikenella corrodens*, and several species not normally associated with periodontal disease in man, such as some of the streptococci.

A summary of the evidence that plaque causes periodontal disease is given in Table 4.1.

4.2 The development of plaque and calculus

Two processes must be differentiated when discussing the development of plaque. One is the development of the plaque flora from birth over a period of many years, a process which depends on transmission of new species to the host with a maturing host response. The other is the re-growth of plaque in a cleaned area, as after oral hygiene procedures, which depends on the reestablishment, at a specific site, of bacteria which are already colonizing other parts of the mouth.

4.2.1 The acquisition of the plaque flora

At birth the oral cavity is sterile, but within a few hours micro-organisms are introduced by transmission from other individuals, and those which are adapted to adhere to the oral mucosa, such as *Streptococcus salivarius*, become established. The oral flora is predominantly streptococcal and rather sparse until the teeth erupt. Then the flora adjusts rapidly to the new environment and organisms adapted to adhere to tooth surfaces form the first dental plaque. A more complex flora becomes well established by about a year and comprises *Streptococcus* sp., *Staphylococcus* sp., *Actinomyces* sp., *Lactobacillus* sp., *Neisseria* sp., and *Veillonella* sp.. New species are continually added throughout childhood, but at puberty there is a marked shift in oral flora as several species implicated in periodontal destruction become established. These changes may be the result of the availability of hormones (which can replace the vitamin K required by some organisms), but concurrent changes in diet and improvement in oral hygiene with age are all reflected in the plaque composition. With the continued eruption of teeth, sites such as the contact areas develop a flora rich in anaerobic bacteria and spirochaetes and these are present in all mouths by adolescence, although the timetable of events is quite variable between individuals. The microbial species which are commonly isolated from the plaque of adults are listed in Table 4.2, together with some of their characteristics.

4.2.2 The re-establishment of supragingival plaque after cleaning

When plaque is removed from the teeth in adults, the cleaned areas are recolonized by bacteria which remain scattered on the tooth surface, in less easily cleaned areas, or from saliva. The bacteria recolonize the surface in a predictable sequence because, as the plaque grows, its structure and internal environment change to favour different species. A clean hydroxyapatite tooth surface is highly reactive and within minutes becomes coated by denatured salivary components, such as glycoprotein, lysozyme and immunoglobulin. A sparse, predominantly

Table 4.2   The more important microbial species in plaque, common isolates, and possible pathogens. Gram staining reflects the structure of the organism wall and, together with any capsule, is an important determinant of susceptibility to different host defence mechanisms. The ecological niche of any oral organism is determined by many factors including its need for, or tolerance of, oxygen and its ability to break down different types of nutrient. Bacteria of early and thin supragingival plaque tend to be aerobic or facultative anaerobes and to ferment carbohydrates such as dietary sugars or salivary glycoproteins. As plaque thickens, filamentous forms and some anaerobes become established. Subgingival plaque contains little oxygen and favours anaerobes which utilize proteins and peptides for energy. Motile bacteria are also much more prominent in subgingival plaque.

Species	Gram stain	Shape	Respiration	Nutritional substrate	Motility
Actinobacillus actinomycetemcomitans	−	cocci/short rod	anaerobic and capnophilic	mostly protein	no
Actinomyces viscosus, A. naeslundii, A. israelii, and *A. odontolyticus*	+	rods and filaments	facultative anaerobe	carbohydrate	no
Corynebacterium matruchotii	+	filament	facultative anaerobe	carbohydrate	no
Branhamella sp.	−	cocci	facultative anaerobe	carbohydrate	no
Capnocytophaga ochracea, C. gingivalis, and *C. sputigena*	−	fusiform rod	anaerobe and capnophilic	protein and carbohydrate	yes
Eikenella corrodens	−	cocci/short rod	microaerophilic	protein	no
Fusobacterium nucleatum	−	slender rod	strict anaerobe	preferentially protein	no
Lactobacillus casei, L. fermentum, L. acidophilus, and *L. plantarum*	+	rods	microaerophilic	carbohydrate	no
Neisseria lactamicus and *N. pharyngis*	−	cocci	facultative anaerobe	carbohydrate	no
Peptococcus sp. and *Peptostreptococcus* sp.	+	cocci	strict anaerobe	protein	no
Porphyromonas gingivalis	−	short rods	strict anaerobe	protein	no
Prevotella melaninogenica, Prev. loeschii, Prev. denticola, Prev. intermedia, and *Prev. oralis*	−	short rods	strict anaerobe	protein and carbohydrate	no
Selenomonas sputigena	−	curved rod	strict anaerobe	protein	yes
Spirochaetes: various poorly defined species other than *Treponema* sp.	−	helical	strict anaerobe	protein	yes
Streptococcus mutans, S. mitis, S. oralis, S. sanguis, S. sobrinus, S. mitior, and *S. milleri*	+	cocci	facultative anaerobe	carbohydrate	no
Treponema denticola, T. macrodentium, T. orale, and *T. vincenti*	−	helical	strict anaerobe	protein	yes
Veillonella alcalescens	−	cocci	strict anaerobe	acids	no
Wollinella recta and *W. succinogenes*	−	curved rod	strict anaerobe	protein	yes

Other less commonly isolated organisms: *Arachnia proprionica, Bifidobacterium dentium, Campylobacter concisus, Eubacterium ingens, Haemophilus parainfluenzae, Haemophilus segnis, Leptotricia buccalis, Micrococcus mucilagenosus, Mycoplasma orale, Mycoplasma salivarium, Propionebacterium acnes, Rothia dentocariosa*, and the protozoan *Entamoeba gingivalis*.

Gram-positive, coccal plaque grows slowly on this organic pellicle (see Fig. 4.2). These bacteria are adapted for adherence and are seeded from the saliva or transferred from other sites by direct contact. Further host components are continually added, including salivary constituents, epithelial cells and neutrophil polymorphonuclear leucocytes (neutrophils), but the seeding of new bacteria is fairly slow and after a few hours the plaque bulk increases by bacterial division instead. After 24 hours plaque becomes visible to the naked eye and individual colonies derived from single bacteria may be seen in areas protected from abrasion. Bacterial numbers double every three hours in this established plaque, which is composed mostly of *Streptococcus sanguis* with a few *Actinomyces* sp.

In undisturbed areas plaque shows increasing complexity as it increases in bulk. Adaptation to adherence becomes less important than competition for the limited nutrients which are available, and over the next few days there is a slow replacement of Gram-positive coccal forms and an increase in anaerobic Gram-negative cocci. Anaerobes become established because oxygen is used up faster than it can diffuse into thick plaque. In mature plaque the competition for nutrients reduces bacterial doubling times to about 24 hours, a much slower rate of division than in young plaque. At about this stage a non-bleeding gingivitis is evident clinically.

In the second half of the first week filamentous forms such as fusiforms and spirochaetes appear and, as the bulk of organisms increases, a bleeding gingivitis is present in most individuals. The total plaque bulk is usually limited by oral hygiene procedures but, in the absence of cleaning, plaque is limited only by abrasion during mastication and may extend to cover tooth crowns and soft tissues. The types of bacteria at these different stages in the recolonization of the tooth surface are shown in Fig. 4.4.

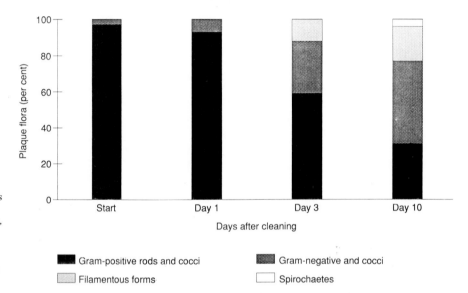

Fig. 4.4 The composition of plaque at various stages during its re-establishment after cleaning. Note how the composition of plaque shows bacterial succession, becoming progressively less coccal and more Gram-negative with time. Note also that this graph shows proportions of the total cultivable flora but that the total number of bacteria increases dramatically with time.

Longitudinal studies of supragingival plaque which extend beyond a few weeks are uncommon. Although there do not appear to be major changes in structure or flora after two weeks, plaque does continue to mature and adapt to the oral environment. The structure of mature plaque is a reflection of its stages of development. Supragingivally and close to the tooth surface is a layer of Gram-positive cocci, the initial colonizers. The plaque becomes progressively more filamentous and complex towards the surface, reflecting the development of a more varied flora. The outermost layer appears to consist mainly of filamentous organisms arranged at right angles to the surface interspersed with many more of the smaller cocci (see Fig. 4.3). A large proportion of mature supragingival plaque, particularly in the deeper layers, consists of dead or metabolically inactive organisms and degraded matrix, but this material is not inert. It is a source of nutrients for some bacterial species and may be as damaging to the gingival tissues as viable plaque.

4.2.3 The development of subgingival plaque

The process by which plaque extends subgingivally as periodontal disease progresses is less easy to investigate than the growth of supragingival plaque, and is thus less well understood. As the gingival crevice deepens, a new environment is created for the plaque flora to colonize. In contrast to exposed tooth surfaces, the crevice is protected from friction, so that attachment and adherence are less important to the flora than in early supragingival plaque. Subgingival plaque accordingly bears little resemblance to adherent supragingival plaque. Although it develops by extension from supragingival plaque, the flora is adapted to a very different environment. The subgingival flora must utilize different nutrients, survive at a lower oxygen concentration, and combat different host defence mechanisms. The initial colonizers are Gram-negative cocci, rods, and spirochaetes and the crevicular or early subgingival plaque may become established as early as four weeks after the onset of clinical gingivitis.

Subgingival plaque becomes more complex with time and the mature plaque in an established pocket consists predominantly of obligate anaerobes or facultative anaerobes such as *Porphyromonas* sp., *Fusobacterium* sp., *Eikenella* sp., *Vibrio* sp., *Selenomonas* sp., and *Capnocytophaga* sp. These do not produce an extracellular matrix and therefore develop into loosely adherent plaque. A large number of species, up to 50 per cent of the total bacteria present, are motile. Despite the absence of matrix, subgingival plaque does retain a recognizable structure because of interbacterial adherence and attachment to the tooth surface and the pocket epithelium. Following periodontal breakdown, the denuded cementum is exposed to the periodontal pocket and is rapidly coated by a pellicle layer derived from crevicular fluid. This pellicle, which often mineralizes, is important in aiding bacterial colonization in a similar way to its saliva-derived supragingival equivalent on enamel.

It is within the periodontal pocket that the maximum microbial diversity is seen and, like supragingival plaque, the subgingival flora is in a continual state of flux. As disease progresses and plaque increases in quantity, it gradually becomes dominated by spirochaetes, motile forms, and Gram-negative rods. At the advancing front of subgingival plaque there are small areas inhabited almost exclusively by single species which represent the equivalent of the individual colonies of bacteria seen in early supragingival plaque. The existence of these microcolonies indicates that subgingival plaque extends apically by the action of a few pioneer bacteria. These are often thought to be motile, but it is possible that they could be driven apically by movements of the teeth and soft tissues. At the base of the pocket there is a narrow plaque-free zone between the top of

Table 4.3 Comparison of supragingival and subgingival plaque

	Supragingival	Subgingival
Matrix	50 per cent matrix	Little or no matrix, plaque is 'unattached'
Flora	Mostly Gram-positive flora, cocci, and short rods	Mostly Gram-negative rods and spirochaetes
Motile bacteria	Few	Common
Anaerobic/aerobic	Aerobic unless thick	Highly anaerobic areas present
Metabolism	Predominantly carbohydrate	Predominantly protein
Species diversity	Little initially, increasing with time	Great

the epithelial attachment and the pioneer bacteria. The size of this potential space varies, but it is usually about one millimetre in width. The significance, if any, of this plaque-free zone is not known. The major differences between subgingival and supragingival plaque are summarized in Table 4.3, and the different plaque floras are summarized in Fig. 4.5.

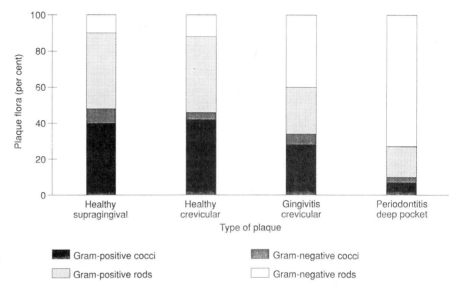

Fig. 4.5 The microbial composition of plaque associated with different degrees of periodontal disease. Note that this graph shows proportions of the total cultivable flora but that the total number of bacteria increases dramatically with disease. It should also be remembered that there is considerable variation between the flora of different patients and different sites within the mouth. This graph shows an average composition.

In the most advanced stages of disease, the top of the pocket gapes open and the environment at the pocket orifice begins to resemble the supragingival environment, so that there is a transition zone where a compact supragingival plaque-like layer extends below the gingival margin on the tooth surface, supporting and merging into the looser or unattached subgingival plaque.

4.2.4 Formation of calculus

Both supragingival and subgingival plaque may mineralize to form calculus. Saliva is supersaturated with calcium phosphate and in susceptible individuals nuclei of mineralization in plaque appear as early as three weeks after re-establishment of plaque. These gradually coalesce and continue to mineralize until calcium phosphate salts account for 70–80 per cent of the weight of the plaque. The nuclei for mineralization are unknown. Although some specific bacterial species promote mineralization *in vitro*, mineralization *in vivo* appears to start in the plaque matrix, before spreading to involve dead bacteria, and is probably related to local pH changes within the plaque. Mineralization proceeds irregularly, so that the calculus has an incremental structure continuous with the dental hard tissues via a layer of calcified pellicle. Unmineralized islands which remain within the calculus probably contain dead bacteria. Supragingival calculus is usually soft, light in colour, and occurs mainly close to salivary duct openings. Subgingival calculus is much harder, dark in colour due to bacterial and blood derived pigments, and occurs at any subgingival site. Calculus is not directly implicated in periodontal disease, but has an indirect effect because it traps plaque close to the gingival tissues.

4.3 Plaque ecology and the structure of plaque

The plaque flora is continually adjusting to environmental changes caused by external influences such as diet, courses of antibiotics, and host defence changes. Different environmental pressures operate at different stages in maturing plaque and the most important are listed in Table 4.4. Initially, large changes in plaque flora (see Fig. 4.4) are seen because the environmental pressures change quickly while the pioneer species are succeeded by a more diverse flora. The mature flora is better able to resist environmental change because of its diversity and, consequently, smaller compensatory adjustments are necessary. Finally, a changing, but relatively stable, plaque ecosystem results from the balance of inter-dependence and antagonism between species and the host defences. This final stable community of bacteria is known as the climax community. The host defences are an important environmental pressure acting on plaque and are discussed in detail in Chapter 5.

Table 4.4 Environmental pressures on plaque bacteria

Adhesion and attachment
    to tooth
    to epithelial cells
    to other bacteria

Nutrient
    substrate availability
    substrate suitability
    inter-dependence for essential nutrients

Population pressure
    bacterial competition for nutrients
    bacteriocins and direct bacterial antagonisms

pH

Oxygen concentration and redox potential

External pressures
    oral hygiene measures
    antibiotics
    host response

4.3.1 Adhesion and attachment

Adhesion and attachment of bacteria to the tooth surface are essential for colonization and to resist the washing effect of saliva and crevicular fluid. The pioneer bacteria in the deepest layers of early plaque, such as *Streptococcus sanguis*, *Streptococcus oralis*, and *Neisseria* sp. possess a glycoprotein coat, specialized appendages, and surface enzymes which enable them to attach to hydroxyapatite, pellicle, matrix, and other bacteria. Once initial bacterial attachment to the tooth has occurred, the production of extracellular matrix and interspecies attachment allows further new species to colonize the early plaque. For example, adhesion between some *Streptococcus* sp. and *Actinomyces* sp. favours establishment of the otherwise non-adherent actinomyces, resulting in the development of a more filamentous plaque. Similar interspecies adhesion is seen between certain filamentous bacteria and streptococci, which coat the filament to produce a structure with the appearance of 'corn on the cob'. This structure is a good example of interspecies adhesion, but, unlike the actinomyces/streptococcal adhesion, appears to be of no significance to the host. Species which are weakly adherent to teeth, such as *Veillonella* sp., become established by adhesion and entrapment in the extracellular matrix produced by the early colonizers and some streptococci are trapped by the aggregating glycoproteins in saliva. Once the early plaque is established, pioneer bacteria such as *Neisseria* sp., which are not adapted to the new environment, are gradually eliminated.

In subgingival plaque, where matrix formation is minimal, it is adherence between bacteria which prevents them being washed from the crevice and determines the structure of subgingival plaque. Attachment to the tooth is essential even subgingivally, and there is always a layer of Gram-positive plaque on the root surface to which the looser Gram-negative plaque adheres.

Adhesion and attachment mechanisms are listed in Table 4.5.

Table 4.5 Adhesion and attachment by plaque bacteria

Adhesion and attachment occur between
  bacteria and cleaned tooth surfaces
  bacteria and pellicle
  bacteria of the same species
  bacteria of different species
  bacteria and matrix

Mechanisms include
  electrostatic attraction
  hydrophobic interaction
  surface enzymes and receptors binding to matrix
  specialized bacterial adhesion structures – fimbriae

4.3.2 Competition for nutrients

Nutrient supply is probably a major environmental pressure on plaque bacteria. Supragingival plaque gains most of its nutrients from saliva rather than directly from the human diet, which has little effect on the structure of plaque unless sucrose intake is very high. Sucrose favours the streptococci which can form both intracellular and extracellular polysaccharide to use as a nutrient supply when sucrose is not present in the mouth. Large amounts of extracellular polysaccharide result in a sticky, tenacious, plaque which is not easily removed by oral hygiene procedures. Early plaque colonizers, such as *S. sanguis* and *S. oralis*, are enzymatically equipped to degrade and metabolize salivary glycoprotein, a more reliable source of nutrient in pellicle and plaque matrix.

Subgingival plaque, by contrast, gains most of its nutrient from the crevicular fluid, a rich and more constant source than is available to supragingival bacteria. The crevicular fluid is rich in protein and contains specific growth factors, such as haem-containing compounds, required by certain micro-organisms. The subgingival microflora is therefore proteolytic and asaccharolytic, secreting enzymes which degrade proteins rather than carbohydrates. The different metabolism of supra- and subgingival plaque thus reflects the nutrients available at each site. The sources of nutrient for plaque are shown in Fig. 4.6.

Plaque contains a complex network of food chains linking all the species into a stable ecosystem. Many species in plaque have the capability to degrade extracellular polysaccharide and, in this way, polymer-producing bacteria provide a constant source of nutrient for their competitors. Nutrients may be incompletely utilized by one species and excreted in a form which can be used by others. For example *Veillonella* sp. can metabolize the acids excreted by the numerous aciduric streptococci. In fact, *Veillonella* sp. are completely dependent on these acids since they do not possess a key glycolytic enzyme. Most such examples relate to individual species, a reflection of the fact that plaque bacteria are highly specific in their requirements for particular nutrients or growth factors. Other examples are the metabolism by *Porphyromonas gingivalis* of vitamin K analogues and succinic acid excreted by Gram-positive organisms, and the metabolism by spirochaetes of growth factors excreted by *Fusobacterium* sp. A large number of such links in food chains are known.

One of the effects of the nutritional dependence in food chains is that individual species do not have to compete directly for nutrient with every other species in plaque, only those with similar metabolic requirements. Competing species use various mechanisms to gain an advantage over competitors. For example, some plaque organisms are inhibited by acid produced by aciduric organisms – the opposite effect to the utilization of such acids noted above. Antagonistic effects may be mediated by secreted factors called bacteriocins. These are usually target-specific but some, such as those secreted by the streptococci, are less so. Many bacteriocins have been described and some are probably active *in vivo*, but they are probably less important than non-specific inhibition by metabolic products such as acids or hydrogen peroxide, which is highly toxic to strict anaerobes.

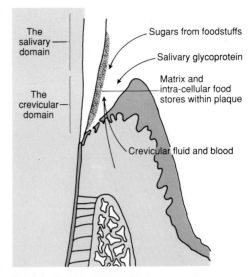

Fig. 4.6 Nutrient sources for plaque bacteria.

4.3.3 Anaerobiosis and the redox potential

An important parameter determining the constituent flora in thick plaque, crevices, and periodontal pockets is the redox potential, a measure of the reducing power of the environment determined by the oxygen concentration and the pH. Although the periodontal pocket itself is not especially anaerobic, oxygen only diffuses in slowly and is continually utilized by both micro-organisms and neutrophils so that deeper pockets have lower redox potentials. When facultative anaerobes become established in plaque they lower the redox potential of the environment by using up oxygen and excreting reducing agents. This renders sites in the depths of subgingival plaque essentially anaerobic and favours colonization by obligate anaerobes. These highly specialized micro-organisms are killed by oxygen so they rarely colonize supragingival plaque. As they cannot use oxygen for respiration they require electron donors and acceptors, such as formate and fumarate, to generate energy. Such compounds are produced in excess by some species so that interdependence based on electron transport compounds probably operates in subgingival plaque in the same way as interdependence on nutrients.

4.3.4 The significance of a stable interdependent plaque ecology

The combined effect of adhesion, nutrient competition, bacterial interdependence, and anaerobiosis is that plaque micro-organisms are integrated into a stable ecosystem. One result is that it is difficult for new species to become established, because the environment is already being exploited maximally by numerous interdependent species, a phenomenon known as population pressure.

Micro-organisms transmitted from other individuals or sites within the mouth are prevented from colonizing a new area of plaque by population pressure, so that the plaque flora differs widely between sites and individuals. The stability of the ecosystem also allows the constituent individual species to resist environmental changes more effectively so that the flora is, in effect, subject to internal homeostatic control.

Another effect of nutrient limitation and bacterial interdependence is that many bacteria grow in sub-optimal conditions, despite the fact that their environment contains rich sources of nutrient. Many plaque species can divide every four hours *in vitro*, when nutrient is in excess, but in plaque they only divide about every 24 hours. This is because external nutrients diffuse poorly into plaque, because of microbial competition, and because many plaque species are fastidious about nutrients. Most species cannot use all the available nutrients, but are limited to certain specific types, so that the rich periodontal environment is able to support a very diverse flora. Nutrient limitation also has a major impact on bacterial structure, metabolism, and antigenicity, all of which are important determinants of bacterial virulence, but unfortunately its effects *in vivo* are poorly understood.

4.4 What makes plaque pathogenic?

Determining why plaque is pathogenic is central to the understanding of periodontal disease, but there is no simple answer. There are many mechanisms by which plaque could damage the host, and more are continually being discovered. Their interrelationships and relative effects in the disease process are not understood. The following sections consider possible pathogenic features of plaque: its physical nature and site, invasion of the tissues by bacteria, release of toxic and inflammatory substances, and the role of specific microbial species.

4.4.1 The physical nature of plaque

Any inflammatory reaction can become chronic if its cause persists, and in the case of gingival inflammation this is plaque. The physical nature of plaque makes its removal difficult, both by the host defences and by oral hygiene measures, and this feature is probably at least as important as any specific microbial factors discussed below.

The build-up of plaque on the oral mucous membranes can be controlled by washing away bacteria with saliva, abrasion by soft tissues and food, or by shedding the surface epithelial cells to which it is attached. Such mechanisms are ineffective on teeth, because plaque is in a relatively protected site and is firmly attached to the host by matrix. Extracellular matrix is produced by a wide variety of bacteria, including *Streptococcus* sp., *Neisseria* sp., *Lactobacillus* sp., *Rothia* sp., and *Actinomyces* sp., but even if the host could somehow eliminate these species, there remains that half of the matrix derived from saliva. The sheer volume of plaque and the rate at which it grows overwhelm the ability of the host defences to remove it physically. Even after toothbrushing individual bacteria remain scattered over the teeth, and these, together with the bacteria in saliva and inaccessible reservoirs of plaque, cannot be completely eliminated. A further handicap to the host defences is the fact that, although plaque is in the mouth, it is effectively outside the body because it is external to the epithelium. The plaque environment is controlled more by the bacteria than the host and is unfavourable to the effective action of most host defence mechanisms. The matrix responsible for attachment also slows the diffusion of host defence factors into plaque and traps a reservoir of bacterial products capable of inhibiting their action.

The net effect of the failure of bacterial shedding, the rapidity of bacterial growth and matrix deposition, and the difficulty of controlling an external flora is that the bacterial mass of plaque becomes relatively large. Unlike most other bacterial infections, the host defences have to deal with a mass of organisms which is big enough to be obvious to the naked eye.

4.4.2 Invasion of the tissues by micro-organisms

Historically it was assumed that periodontal disease was the result of bacterial invasion of the periodontium and bone. The convincing demonstration of bacteria within the periodontal tissues is, however, technically difficult and has been plagued by artefacts. Meticulous techniques show that micro-organisms do penetrate into the tissues, but not frequently enough for invasion to be considered as the major cause of periodontal disease.

Invasion would be expected to exacerbate tissue damage. However, plaque bacteria are commensal rather than pathogenic in nature and would be expected to be eliminated rapidly from the tissues, either by the host defences or, in the case of anaerobes, to be killed by oxygen. A few species, such as *P. gingivalis*, can disseminate after subcutaneous inoculation into animals, but they do not appear to do so when introduced into the oral cavity. Most plaque bacteria in the tissues are probably not invasive in the true sense of the word, because they are not adapted to survive and divide within the host and cannot colonize the tissues. Tissue penetration is probably an effect of disease, the result of pocket ulceration and tooth movement rather than the virulence of the bacteria. The flora which does penetrate the tissues appears to consist of Gram-negatives and spirochaetes, reflecting the species found in deep pockets, and their numbers are related to the severity of disease. Some studies have reported that invading bacteria seem to elicit little host response and that bacteria are only occasionally seen within phagocytes. It is possible that bacterial penetration is an important factor in bursts of active or very advanced disease, but its importance is not yet clear.

4.4.3 Soluble factors derived from bacteria

Plaque bacteria are commensal and remain limited to the pocket, and so it is widely hypothesized that soluble bacterial products might penetrate the host tissues. Such soluble factors, or the host reaction to them, might cause the tissue damage characteristic of periodontal disease. As discussed in Chapter 2 the junctional epithelium is relatively permeable and this may allow soluble products to pass into the tissues as well as allowing host defence factors easy access to the crevice, but the extent to which bacterial factors can penetrate the tissues is not known. Many factors capable of damaging the host have been described and the most important are listed in Table 4.6, but whether these compounds cause damage *in vivo* is not known.

Despite considerable effort, there is little good direct evidence to show the presence of bacterial factors (as opposed to whole bacteria) in the tissues because of technical difficulties. Penetration of soluble factors is resisted first by the junctional epithelium (see pp. 20–1), but this is relatively permeable and becomes

Table 4.6 Possible pathogenic bacterial products

Factor	Produced by	How produced	Effects
Leukotoxin	*A. actinomycetemcomitans*	Secreted and in membrane vesicles	Specific inhibition of neutrophils and monocyte/macrophages
Lipopolysaccharide (endotoxins)	Gram-negative bacteria	Outer membrane component released on growth and lysis and in membrane vesicles	Activates complement Activates macrophages and neutrophils Activates bone resorption Polyclonal B cell activator Immunological adjuvant
Lipoteichoic acid (LTA)	Gram-positive bacteria	Cell wall component released on growth and lysis	Less potent than endotoxins Activates bone resorption
Actinomyces 'resorbing factor'	*Actinomyces* sp.	The equivalent of LTA in *Actinomyces* sp.	Potency and effects as LTA
Capsular material	Some Gram-positive and some Gram-negative bacteria	Outer layer of carbohydrate and hydrophobic peptide on cell wall	Enables bacteria to resist phagocytosis Prevents complement activation Some are potent activators of bone resorption
Muramyl dipeptide	Gram-positive and -negative bacteria	Dipeptide component of cell wall degradation product and secreted	Polyclonal B cell activator Immunological adjuvant May also suppress immune response by action on T cell Activates bone resorption
Short chain fatty acids	Various bacteria	Excretory product of metabolism	Inhibits chemotaxis and killing by neutrophils
Dextrans	*Streptococcus* sp., *Actinomyces* sp., *Lactobacillus* sp., *Neisseria* sp., and a few others	Extracellular polysaccharide matrix of plaque	Polyclonal B cell activator Immunological adjuvant

Hydrolytic enzymes:
  Hyaluronidase
  Collagenases
  Proteases
  Phosphatases
  Phospholipases
	Many bacterial species and the spirochaetes	Secreted extracellularly
		Membrane vesicles in some species
			Degrade tissue components, such as:
			  collagen and connective tissue ground substance
			  immunoglobulins (some enzymes degrade only some classes)
			  complement components

Butyric/propionic acids, indole, ammonia	Anaerobic bacteria and spirochaetes	Secreted extracellularly	Toxic and inhibitory effects on many host cells
Reducing agents, mercaptans and H_2S	Anaerobic proteolytic bacteria	Secreted extracellularly	Increase epithelial permeability Inhibit immune function and fibroblasts

ulcerated in disease (see p. 35). Once the gingiva become inflamed, the flow of crevicular fluid washes soluble products out of the crevice, but the flow is very variable between sites and is almost absent at some (see pp. 34–5). The combination of these circumstances probably does allow tiny amounts of bacterial products into the tissues. The best evidence for this is that soluble antigens applied to the gingival crevice stimulate antibody production in lymph nodes and periodontal tissues (although as noted on p. 19 this can also occur through the action of Langerhans cells in the oral gingival epithelium without antigen entering the tissues). Antibodies against plaque antigens are generated in disease (see Chapter 5) and levels correlate with severity, suggesting that plaque components probably penetrate the tissues more easily in advanced disease.

Many damaging soluble compounds are either known or presumed to be present in plaque and are often described as toxins though, unlike the classical toxins, they act locally on the disease process, rather than at remote sites. Some are of the endotoxin type, components of bacteria released in large amounts after death and smaller quantities during life, while others are exotoxin-like and are continually secreted during life. Some do not fall neatly into either category. Their actions may be divided into direct toxic effects on host cells, activation or interference with inflammatory and immunological processes, enzymic activities capable of degrading host components, and some whose mechanisms of action are unknown.

Bacterial products with direct toxic effects

Bacterial endotoxins are potent factors produced by all Gram-negative bacteria and have been proposed to be virulence factors in periodontal disease. They are capable of many actions including activation of the complement and coagulation cascades, macrophage and lymphocyte activation, degranulation of neutrophils, and stimulation of bone resorption, and are also chemotactic and antigenic (see Chapter 5). Some of these effects may be mediated by stimulation of interleukin-1 secretion by host cells. Although many other factors also stimulate some of these responses, endotoxin is unusual in its ability to stimulate almost the entire range of host responses in inflammation.

Endotoxins consist principally of lipopolysaccharides which are released from the outer layers of the cell wall during growth and after lysis. After release, lipopolysaccharide is coupled to protein to form the final endotoxin, but it is the lipopolysaccharide itself which is the biologically active part of the toxin and its structure varies between bacterial species. All lipopolysaccharides contain Lipid A, a core or C polysaccharide, and an outer or O polysaccharide (see Fig. 4.7) and slight differences in these constituents affect the relative potency of the endotoxin. Many endotoxins from plaque bacteria, notably those from *P. gingivalis*, are markedly less toxic than those from *Escherichia coli* and *Salmonella typhi*, which are responsible for the life-threatening condition known as endotoxic shock. Endotoxin derived from plaque is still, however, a potent mediator of many inflammatory reactions and it is released continually in membrane vesicles from organisms such as *P. gingivalis* and *A. actinomycetemcomitans* and in a soluble form from many other organisms. It is estimated that there are 100 nanograms of endotoxin in an average person's dental plaque, enough to produce marked systemic effects if it all entered the tissues at once.

The best example of an exotoxin-like toxin secreted by a plaque bacterium is *A. actinomycetemcomitans* leucotoxin, which is directed at neutrophils and monocytes and causes plasma membrane damage (see pp. 61–2). The fact

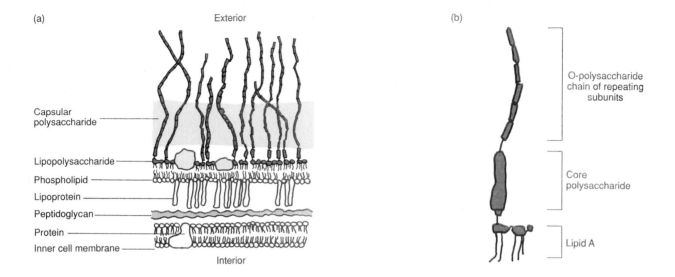

Fig. 4.7 The structure of bacterial endotoxin and the Gram-negative cell wall showing other components which can be virulence determinants.

that leucotoxic strains correlate better with disease than non-leucotoxic strains suggests that the toxin may be active *in vivo*. Other species secrete a number of factors described as toxic for certain types of host cell, but these are as yet poorly defined.

Most plaque bacteria produce acids as metabolic products and some have specific toxic effects independent of their acidity. Some short chain fatty acids, especially succinic and butyric acids, inhibit various neutrophil functions.

Bacterial products which affect host mechanisms

Plaque also contains a number of unrelated compounds which, at least *in vitro*, have effects on inflammatory and immunological mechanisms. Many bacterial products are recognized as foreign by the host and elicit an immune response, with either the production of specific antibodies or the activation of cell mediated immunity. In addition, some modulate immune reactions. Plaque extracts and some specific plaque products have adjuvant activity, enhancing the immune response to other molecules. Other bacterial products, known as polyclonal B cell activators, stimulate antibody production by plasma cells in a non-specific, antigen-independent manner. The antibody produced is not directed against the activator but against whichever antigen each individual B cell is programmed to recognize (see pp. 83–5). Mechanisms such as these could reduce the efficiency of the immunological response in periodontal disease and may also worsen bystander damage (the random damage of adjacent tissues) resulting from immunological mechanisms. Other host processes may be activated by bacterial products. A number of factors have been shown to be potent stimulators of bone resorption *in vitro* and these are discussed in Chapter 6. Many products have been reported to activate macrophages and neutrophils and to fix and activate complement. The number of plaque products which have been reported to interfere with host defence mechanisms is thus very large, but the number which are important *in vivo* is unknown.

Enzyme mediated mechanisms

Plaque bacteria produce many enzymes which may digest components of host tissues or interfere with their homeostasis and repair. Among such enzymes are collagenase, hyaluronidase and a number of proteases which break down immunoglobulins, complement, and other host proteins. Some are rather non-specific in their action while others have a narrow spectrum of activity. Many have been described and their role is probably to provide nutrients in the crevicular environment. If these enzymes are to have any pathological significance they must retain their activity within plaque and possibly the tissues, but most would be quickly degraded or inactivated by the many other proteases and enzyme inhibitors present in crevicular fluid and the tissues. Whether any retain significant activity *in vivo* is unknown.

4.4.4 Specific pathogens within plaque

The specific and non-specific plaque hypotheses

Although the amount of plaque present correlates well with disease severity in epidemiological studies, it correlates poorly in individual patients. Many patients have considerable plaque deposits, but only a minority suffer destructive periodontal disease – and even then often in only a few sites. This paradox might be explained by the specific plaque hypothesis, which proposes that destructive periodontal disease is the result of specific microbial pathogens in plaque. Such a theory is attractive, since it can explain the wide variations in disease in terms of the variability which is known to occur in the composition of plaque. The concept of the specific plaque hypothesis is illustrated by making a comparison with dental caries, where specific pathogens are well recognized. Although the specific plaque hypothesis remains unproven for periodontal disease, it is a useful and valid concept and a number of species have been proposed as specific pathogens. However, there are many damaging factors in plaque which are derived either from several species or from plaque as a whole. It may not be necessary to postulate the presence of specific pathogens and many workers prefer the concept known as the non-specific plaque hypothesis. This states that it is the total bulk of plaque which determines its pathogenicity, rather than the individual species within it.

It is the non-specific plaque hypothesis which forms the basis for virtually all current strategies for treatment and prevention, which rely on the principle of reducing plaque levels to a minimum. Proponents of the specific theory point out that non-specifically reducing plaque levels also maintains a more aerobic, and therefore possibly less pathogenic, flora. The non-specific hypothesis is successful as a rationale for treatment, but it does tend to imply that all patients must maintain a high standard of oral hygiene to prevent tooth loss. The identification of specific pathogens would allow detection of the relatively small number of patients at special risk and enable them to be treated more vigorously, and might lead to treatments targeted at specific bacteria. The search is on for possible pathogens and the literature contains many reports of bacterial species and their supposed virulence factors, but isolation and identification of periodontal pathogens is an extremely difficult task. Some of the reasons for this are considered below.

How can periodontal pathogens be identified?

It is generally assumed that periodontal pathogens are likely to form a major part of the plaque flora during active disease, that numbers will correlate with disease activity at individual sites, and that they will be absent from healthy sites. To demonstrate this, it is necessary to identify species in plaque at individual sites and then show that those sites, but not others, suffer periodontal breakdown. Unfortunately, we are currently unable to determine from a single observation whether disease is progressing, regressing, or remaining static at a single site and the chances of a single sample being taken when the disease is active are small. Most microbiological studies can therefore only associate species with specific signs such as bleeding or bone loss. A few studies have monitored the flora at a single site over a long period which included periods of active disease, but such studies have not yet been successful at identifying pathogens.

The complexity of plaque and the limitations of microbiological culture studies also make the identification of periodontal pathogens difficult. There are about 10^8 micro-organisms per mm^3 in plaque, each site containing a different selection from over 200 species of bacteria, yeasts, mycoplasmas, and protozoa. The flora varies considerably between individuals, between sites in any one individual, and also with time, and – even with the most advanced anaerobic sampling techniques – only about 70 per cent of plaque bacteria can be grown. The problems of identifying a small number of pathogens from plaque are illustrated by a study of adult periodontal disease in which 60 diseased sites yielded 171 plaque species, 74 of them unclassifiable. In the subgingival plaque, 37 species were associated with health and 99 with disease. Twenty eight species were considered potential pathogens but, unfortunately, many have been reported in other studies as being present in healthy sites. The most recent methods, such as fluorescent antibody binding and DNA probes, can detect very small numbers of bacteria within plaque and hold promise for the future, but have not yet been applied to large scale studies.

The final problem in identifying periodontal pathogens is one of interpretation. If a pathogen could be clearly associated with disease progression it would still not be possible to say whether the association was causative or the result of a change induced in the plaque by the disease process itself. It would be desirable to show that a pathogenic species appeared or multiplied in plaque just before a burst of active disease.

In conclusion, microbiological studies have proposed that certain bacterial species are periodontal pathogens, but their identification is fraught with conceptual and practical difficulties. The best known of these pathogens are discussed below, together with some of their possible pathogenic mechanisms.

Possible periodontal pathogens

Although we cannot prove a causative association between specific microbial species and destructive periodontal disease, there are a number of species whose presence has been correlated with severe disease or specific features such as gingival bleeding. A consensus view that these species are important has emerged because they have been correlated with disease in several studies. Further evidence of pathogenicity has been sought for these species and many possible pathogenic mechanisms have been described *in vitro*. Even though such evidence may appear strong, it should always be remembered that it is only circumstantial. The possible pathogens described below have an impressive array of potential virulence factors, but many factors are also associated with non-pathogenic species as well. A good example to illustrate this point is *Capnocytophaga* sp., a species which produces a lipopolysaccharide which triggers bone resorption, several extracellular proteases, and capsular material which inhibits neutrophil function. Despite such potential virulence factors, *Capnocytophaga* sp. seems to be found at healthy sites and is not, therefore, a periodontal pathogen. Consequently it seems that many so-called pathogenic or virulence mechanisms may actually perform other functions. For instance, many potential pathogens secrete proteases which are capable of degrading immunoglobulin and complement, and it is often assumed that this protects them from the host defences. In fact, most of the subgingival microflora produce such proteases, because their main source of nutrient is the crevicular fluid, which is rich in immunoglobulin and complement. Such proteases may indeed be important for virulence, not because they attack the host but because they allow some bacteria to colonize the periodontal pocket more effectively.

Possible pathogens in gingivitis

The evidence that specific pathogens have a role in gingivitis is mainly derived from the study of experimental gingivitis, but this model may not be relevant to a longstanding gingivitis where the plaque is considerably more complex. In the experimental gingivitis model, gingival inflammation with bleeding appears 10–21 days following cessation of oral hygiene measures. At this time the plaque is fairly simple, with *Actinomyces* sp. – especially *Actinomyces viscosus* – just becoming established. This finding has led to the proposal that *A. viscosus* is a specific pathogen for gingivitis. Other evidence supporting a role for *A. viscosus* as a specific pathogen comes from monoinfection in animals, although here it causes a severe destructive periodontitis rather than gingivitis.

However, although *A. viscosus* used to be thought a significant pathogen, this is no longer the case. More recent studies have shown it to be a common constituent of plaque associated with healthy gingiva. During experimental gingivitis it appears several days before the onset of bleeding, but is only one of a large number of species which correlate with bleeding. Plaque before, during, and just after the onset of gingivitis is very similar and it is now accepted that gingivitis is microbiologically non-specific. Onset of bleeding is probably related to the plaque mass and the time in contact with the gingiva, rather than the organisms it contains.

Possible pathogens in periodontitis

Although gingivitis is a relatively non-specific inflammatory response to plaque, periodontitis could, on the other hand, be associated with specific bacterial species. Unfortunately, the task of identifying specific pathogens in periodontal disease is considerably more difficult than in gingivitis. Unlike gingivitis, where plaque accumulates evenly and inflammation occurs all along the gingival margin, destructive periodontal disease develops unpredictably in a few sites, all of which can have widely differing flora. Despite these difficulties, good evidence has now been accumulated to implicate several species and strains in the pathogenesis of disease. The best known are listed in Table 4.7 and are discussed below.

Porphyromonas gingivalis

This species, previously known as *Bacteroides gingivalis*, is a strictly anaerobic Gram-negative rod which produces a black pigment. It is probably the species most strongly associated with adult periodontitis and rapidly progressive disease in man and also causes periodontal destruction in gnotobiotic animals. A variety of possible virulence mechanisms have been identified. It has a carbohydrate capsule on its outer surface which prevents opsonization by complement and inhibits phagocytosis and killing by neutrophils. Its lipopolysaccharide is not very toxic, but it inhibits chemotaxis and killing by leucocytes. Toxins affecting epithelial cells and fibroblasts are also secreted. More importantly, *P. gingivalis* possesses the widest spectrum of tissue degrading enzymes of the proposed

Table 4.7 Possible specific periodontal pathogens

Bacterial species	Evidence	Proposed virulence factors
Actinomyces viscosus	Correlates approximately with the onset of bleeding in gingivitis Causes periodontal destruction in gnotobiotic animals	Surface coating Actinomyces bone resorbing factor
Porphyromonas gingivalis	Correlates with adult periodontitis, rapidly progressive disease and ANUG Causes periodontal destruction in gnotobiotic animals	Activates complement poorly Resists phagocytosis and killing by neutrophils Capsular material 'Toxic' effects on epithelial cells and fibroblasts Lipopolysaccharide inhibits chemotaxis Enzymes degrade immunoglobulins, complement, collagen, connective tissue ground substances Membrane vesicles
Actinobacillus actinomycetemcomitans	Correlates with juvenile periodontitis and rapidly progressive periodontitis, and less well with adult periodontitis Causes periodontal destruction in gnotobiotic animals	Leucotoxin (toxic for neutrophils and monocytes) Toxic effects on epithelial cells and fibroblasts Capsular material Activates complement poorly Resists phagocytosis Lipopolysaccharide, active for bone resorption Some hydrolytic enzymes, collagenase Forms membrane vesicles May be tissue 'invasive'
Fusobacterium nucleatum	Correlates with ANUG and rapidly progressive periodontal disease Causes periodontal destruction in gnotobiotic animals	Potent lipopolysaccharide Excretes butyric acid Synergic with *P. gingivalis* in culture
Spirochaetes	Associated with ANUG May correlate with adult and rapidly progressing periodontal disease	Hydrolytic enzymes, collagenase Unusual excretory products Some produce membrane vesicles Virulence factors very difficult to determine *in vitro*
Prevotella intermedia	Correlates with ANUG and, less well, with adult periodontal disease	Capsular material Resists phagocytosis Lipopolysaccharide Toxic effect on epithelial cells Secretion of some hydrolytic enzymes
Bacteroides gracilis *Bacteroides ureolyticus* *Campylobacter concisus* *Eikenella corrodens* *Wollinella recta*	All may be associated with disease *Campylobacter* sp., *Eikenella* sp., and *Wolinella* sp. cause periodontal destruction in gnotobiotic animals	Various described
Capnocytophaga species	Have been associated with juvenile periodontitis and adult periodontal disease Now also known to be present in healthy sites Causes periodontal destruction in gnotobiotic animals	Lipopolysaccharide activates bone resorption Enzymes degrade immunoglobulin Capsular material Resists phagocytosis and inhibits chemotaxis

periodontal pathogens. Proteases which degrade immunoglobulin, complement, collagen, and hyaluronic acid appear to be likely virulence determinants, but fibrinolysins, phospholipases, and many others are secreted. A feature of this species is the formation of membrane vesicles (30–150nm in diameter), which are shed in very large numbers and carry with them the secreted protease. Their small size may enable them to pass into the tissues. *P. gingivalis* requires haem compounds for growth and is able to obtain them from haemoglobin in blood. This may explain the fact that during experimental gingivitis it becomes established at about the time that gingival bleeding occurs. It also requires vitamin K or its analogues which, as noted earlier, can be supplied by other species in plaque.

Prevotella intermedia

Prevotella intermedia (previously known as *Bacteroides intermedius*) is a black pigmented Gram-negative bacterium which can ferment both carbohydrate and proteins and is thus equally at home in supra- and subgingival plaque. The presence of *Prev. intermedia* correlates with acute necrotizing ulcerative gingivitis and with adult periodontal disease. Like *P. gingivalis*, this species resists phagocytosis, probably by virtue of its capsule, but there is considerable variation between strains and genotypes. The lipopolysaccharide contains unusual fatty acids and is thought to have marked effects on immune and bone cells. A toxin acting on epithelial cells is secreted by some strains, but *Prev. intermedia* does not secrete the range of hydrolytic enzymes of *P. gingivalis*. It is not a constant species in plaque and it is also found in the gastrointestinal tract, which makes the relevance of serum antibody levels to periodontal disease difficult to interpret.

Actinobacillus actinomycetemcomitans

A. actinomycetemcomitans is a Gram-negative non-motile coccoid bacillus whose presence in the periodontal pocket is correlated with juvenile periodontitis, rapidly progressive periodontitis, and adult periodontitis in man and animals. It is perhaps the best candidate to be a specific pathogen, especially in localized juvenile periodontitis. *A. actinomycetemcomitans* is also found associated with many other human infections including urinary tract infections, meningitis, and osteomyelitis.

Several virulence factors are reported, amongst which the leucotoxin is probably the most important. Leucotoxin is one of a family of cytolysins which include *E. coli* α-haemolysin and *Pasteurella* sp. haemolytic toxin, but it is directed against neutrophils and monocytes, rather than erythrocytes. The toxin therefore has the potential to interfere with both non-specific and immunological host defences. It is potent, but acts relatively slowly, causing cell swelling and leakage, so that when tested *in vitro* neutrophils can still kill the bacteria for a time in the presence of the toxin. Not all strains are leucotoxic and disease correlates better with the presence of toxin-producing strains and may vary with levels of specific antibody which can neutralize the toxin. Distinct toxins affecting epithelial cells and fibroblasts are also secreted.

A. actinomycetemcomitans also possesses a capsule which confers complement and phagocytosis resistance, fimbriae, a lipopolysaccharide with extremely potent bone resorbing activity and the ability to interfere with neutrophil function, and a variety of tissue destructive enzymes including a collagenase. Like *P. gingivalis*, it also forms membrane vesicles which carry some of these activities into the surrounding environment.

A. actinomycetemcomitans is one of the bacteria which has been found within the periodontal tissues, but it is not clear whether this reflects an intrinsic ability to invade tissues and colonize them in the classical sense. *A. acti-nomycetemcomitans* is certainly capable of causing tissue infections at other sites in the body, but is most commonly part of a mixed infection, often actinomycosis. Antibiotic therapy is sometimes used for juvenile periodontitis, and tetracycline is the drug of choice because strains resistant to penicillin, metronidazole, and erythromycin are frequent.

Fusobacterium nucleatum

Three subspecies of this Gram-negative rod have been identified; *F. nucleatum, Fusobacterium fusiforme,* and *Fusobacterium polymorphum. F. nucleatum* is now regarded as an important periodontal pathogen, particularly subspecies nucleatum, which is most commonly associated with diseased sites in acute necrotizing ulcerative gingivitis and rapidly progressive periodontal disease. Virulence of this species has been attributed to its potent lipopolysaccharide and the production of butyric acid as a metabolic end product. The species lacks any major hydrolytic enzyme activity apart from a haemolysin, but may act synergistically in mixed culture with *P. gingivalis* to increase protease secretion. Adhesins on its surface enable *F. nucleatum* to adhere to epithelial cells, leucocytes, erythrocytes, fibroblasts, and other bacterial species. These properties may be important in early colonization by this species, particularly in early subgingival plaque.

Spirochaetes

Spirochaetes are motile spiral-shaped micro-organisms bearing flagella. In advanced disease they comprize up to 50 per cent of the observable bacteria in plaque, and high numbers have been associated with acute necrotizing ulcerative gingivitis, where they invade the superficial tissues, and, less well, with adult and rapidly progressing periodontal disease. They do not appear to be associated with localized juvenile periodontitis, in which few spirochaetes are present. Unfortunately, these disease associations have proved difficult to investigate because all spirochaetes are difficult to isolate, grow, and identify. Which spirochaete species are associated with disease is still unclear. There are two important oral species, *Treponema denticola* and *Treponema vincentii*, both of which produce potent hydrolytic enzymes including collagenases, proteinases, and peptidases. Both species produce a lipopolysaccharide of the low virulence type. *T. denticola* produces extracellular membrane vesicles which have protease and haemagglutinating activity. Spirochaetes also release unusual metabolic end products, such as indole, hydrogen sulphide, and ammonia, which are potentially toxic to host cells and some bacteria, but which other bacteria may utilize.

Other motile and Gram-negative rods

There are several other Gram-negative bacteria with unusual properties which are correlated with disease, including *Campylobacter concisus, Wollinella recta* (motile), *Bacteroides gracilis* (motile by a slow twitching movement), *Bacteroides ureolyticus,* and *Eikenella corrodens* (corrodes the surface of agar plates). All are commonly isolated from gingivitis and periodontal pockets and are possibly associated with the advancing front of the plaque, perhaps because of their motility. In general these species neither ferment carbohydrate nor utilize proteins as energy sources, but exploit substances such as formate, and other electron donors, or fumarate, and other electron acceptors. Thus they may play an important part in the complex nutritional network of gingival ecosystem, although they may not be directly pathogenic. Apart from *Eikenella* sp. all produce succinate, a metabolic end product which can be utilized by other bacteria such as *P. gingivalis*.

Capnocytophaga species

Capnocytophaga are micro-aerophilic Gram-negative rods which move by a gliding action and produce carotenoid pigments. There are three species, *Capnocytophaga ochracea*, *Capnocytophaga sputigena*, and *Capnocytophaga gingivalis*, of which *C. ochracea* (formerly *Bacteroides ochracea*) is the most extensively studied. It has been linked with juvenile periodontitis and adult periodontal disease by culture studies and causes disease in animal models. A number of virulence factors have been proposed to support this association. *C. ochracea* produces a lipoplysaccharide with bone resorbing activity but low complement fixing activity, extracellular proteases which degrade immunoglobulins, and copious capsular material which inhibits phagocytosis and chemotaxis. More recent studies have shown that C. ochracea is often isolated from healthy sites and it should not be regarded as a significant pathogen. It is included here to illustrate the point that these possible virulence mechanisms only provide circumstantial evidence for pathogenicity, rather than clear proof.

Multiple pathogen theories

The number of bacterial species implicated in periodontal disease is considerable and it seems likely that, unless totally new pathogenic species are isolated, the search for a single key pathogen is unlikely to be fruitful. On the other hand, many bacteria are associated with healthy sites, so the non-specific plaque hypothesis is unlikely to be absolutely correct either. It has therefore been proposed that a small number of interacting species might cause destructive disease. This theory, intermediate between the specific and non-specific theories is a rational one, but identifying the combinations of pathogens which are important is likely to be difficult.

The best example of synergy in a periodontal infection is acute necrotizing ulcerative gingivitis in which spirochaetes and *Fusobacterium* sp. invade the tissues, usually when the host resistance is lowered (*Prev. intermedia* and *P. gingivalis* are also strongly associated, see pp. 59–61). It is likely that other synergistic interactions occur subgingivally in adult periodontitis and studies have identified groups of organisms which correlate better with disease than single species alone. Such groups include *F. nucleatum* with *P. gingivalis* and *Eikenella* sp., *P. gingivalis* with *W. recta* and small spirochaetes, and the combination of *P. intermedia*, *E. corrodens*, and *F. nucleatum*. The virulence of such combinations has usually been tested in non-oral sites. When plaque is injected into the tissues it results in an infection in which Gram-negative anaerobes predominate. If *P. gingivalis*, black pigmented rods, or *Fusobacterium* sp. are present the infections become necrotic. Using such models, synergy can be demonstrated between *P. gingivalis* and various Gram-positive bacteria, between *Klebsiella* sp. (which provide growth factors), *F. nucleatum* and spirochaetes, and between *P. gingivalis* and *F. nucleatum* (enhanced proteolytic activity). However, the relevance of these synergistic interactions to periodontal disease is unclear.

One group of organisms which has received particular attention is the motile organisms, partly because they may be easily identified at the chairside by dark ground microscopy. Although motile organisms are associated with disease in cross sectional studies of the population, a simple correlation is not seen in individual patients or individual periodontal pockets. Unfortunately the technique is rather non-specific and cannot differentiate between the numerous motile species in plaque, most of which are Gram-negative rods or spirochaetes. The method may be useful for measuring plaque maturity to monitor treatment, but it has proved to be of no diagnostic or predictive value.

Multiple pathogen theories are generally concerned with only a few microbial species, usually from amongst the organisms discussed on pp. 59–63. However, it is possible that the number of species necessary to form pathogenic plaque is much larger because of the complex synergistic interactions necessary to form a stable plaque ecology. From an ecological perspective, it could be argued that no individual bacterial species is a specific pathogen, but rather that certain species fill essential ecological niches within plaque, which then becomes pathogenic because of its overall metabolism and stable ecosystem in the pocket. Investigation of this much more complex theory is in its infancy.

Specific pathogens – conclusions

Numerous specific pathogens have been proposed as causes of periodontal disease. The evidence for each is circumstantial and is based on association with disease and *in vitro* studies because definitive investigations are extremely difficult to perform. An unsuspected pathogen might still exist in the 25 per cent of the flora which cannot be cultivated or identified and there has been little investigation into viruses and mycoplasmas in this context.

We have no good criteria to identify periodontal pathogens and the specific plaque hypothesis cannot, in any case, be proven by microbiological culture studies alone. Microbiological studies have proposed a limited number of potential pathogens (see Table 4.7) on the basis of a large body of well researched data, and a new hypothesis is now emerging. Gingivitis appears to be a non-specific phenomenon related to plaque accumulation. Destructive periodontal disease may be the result of shifts in plaque flora, which could be transient, during which groups of potentially pathogenic bacteria form plaque which has a pathogenic ecology. This theory is intermediate between the non-specific and specific plaque hypotheses, neither of which appears to apply directly to destructive periodontitis. What allows a pathogenic plaque to form and stabilize remains unknown, but alterations in both the host response to plaque bacteria and the ecological interactions between bacteria are likely to be important.

4.5 Summary

1. Human and animal studies have shown bacterial plaque to be the cause of periodontitis.

2. Plaque is an extremely complex structure, comprising a highly variable flora, and a matrix composed of host and bacterial derived components. Its ecology makes detailed investigation difficult.

3. Plaque could be pathogenic because:

    (i)   it is outside the tissues and difficult for the host defences to deal with;
    (ii) it releases a very large number of soluble factors including enzymes, toxins and metabolic products which are known to be toxic, inflammatory or antigenic;
    (iii) it may contain certain pathogenic microbial species.

4. Gingivitis seems to be a non-specific reaction to plaque accumulation.

5. In periodontal disease:

    (i)   clinical features such as bleeding or deep pocketing correlate well with the presence of certain species in plaque, but these species can also occur in health;

(ii) specific pathogen(s) may be responsible for tissue destruction. No single proven pathogen has yet been identified;

(iii) some potential pathogens possess possible virulence factors which may either allow them to compete for nutrient or disable the host defences in the pocket environment;

(iv) tissue damage may also be caused by combinations of bacteria;

(v) pathogenicity may be related to the ecology and metabolism of the plaque present, rather than to the individual species within it.

6. It is not possible to explain periodontal disease in terms of microbiology alone. As in any disease, host factors affecting the resistance to plaque and bacteria are important. Such factors are the subject of the following chapter.

4.6 Further reading

Note that *Porphyromonas gingivalis* was classified as *Bacteroides gingivalis* when many of these papers were written, and that some refer to *Actinobacillus actinomycetemcomitans* as *Haemophilus actinomycetemcomitans*.

Oral microbiology of plaque and plaque ecology

Marsh, P.D. and Martin, M. (1984). *Oral Microbiology* (2nd edn). (Van Nostrand Reinhold, London).
— *An excellent text for basic plaque microbiology, although several bacterial species have been reclassified and renamed since it was written.*

Marsh, P.D. (1990). The microbiology of periodontal disease in *Periodontics, a practical approach* (ed. J.B. Kieser). (Wright, London).
— *An up to date definitive review of plaque microbiology, particularly its ecological aspects.*

Gingivitis

Löe, H., Theilade, E., and Jensen, S. (1965). Experimental gingivitis in man. *J. Periodontol.* **36**, 177–87.
Theilade, E., Wright, W., Jensen, S., and Löe, H. (1965). Experimental gingivitis in man II. A longitudinal clinical and bacteriological study investigation. *J. Periodont. Res.* **1**, 1–13.
— *Two classic studies of experimental gingivitis and its microbiology.*

Loesche, W.J. and Syed, S.A. (1978). Bacteriology of human experimental gingivitis: effect of plaque and gingivitis score. *Infect. Immun.* **21**, 830–9.

Periodontitis

Theilade, E. (1986). The non-specific theory in microbial aetiology of inflammatory periodontal diseases. *J. Clin. Periodontol.* **13**, 905–11.
Slots, J. (1986). Bacterial specificity in adult periodontitis. A summary of recent work. *J. Clin. Periodontol.* **13**, 912–91.
— *Two papers proposing the opposite points of view of the non-specific and specific plaque theories.*

Moore, W. (1987). Microbiology of periodontal disease. *J. Periodont. Res.* **22**, 335–41.
— *A review of the search for specific pathogens.*

Socransky, S.S., Haffajee, A.D., Smith, G.L., and Dzink, J.L. (1987). Difficulties encountered in the search for the aetiologic agents of destructive periodontal diseases. *J. Clin. Periodontol.* **14**, 588–93.

Maiden, M.F.J., Carman R.J., Curtis, M.A., Gillett, I.R., Griffiths, G.S., Sterne, J.A.C., *et al.* (1990). Detection of high risk groups and individuals for periodontal diseases: laboratory markers based on the microbiological analysis of subgingival plaque. *J. Clin. Periodontol.* **17**, 1–13.

— *Two papers discussing the technical and conceptual difficulties of identifying periodontal pathogens and applying the findings to detect patients at high risk of periodontitis.*

Slots, J. and Genco, R.J. (1984). Microbial pathogenicity. Black pigmented *Bacteroides* species, *Capnocytophaga* species, and *Actinobacillus actinomycetemcomitans* in human periodontal disease: virulence factors in colonization, survival, and tissue destruction. *J. Dent. Res.* **63**, 412–21.

— *A review of evidence to support a pathogenic role for these organisms.*

5 Host defences against microbial plaque

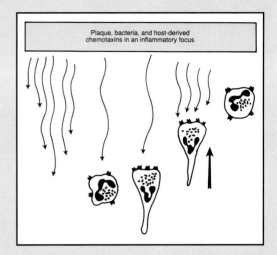

Plaque, bacteria, and host-derived chemotaxins in an inflammatory focus

This chapter describes the role of host defences in the pathogenesis of periodontal disease. The functions of the host defences are to keep bacteria and their products out of the periodontium and to destroy any which succeed in entering the tissues. The first level of host defence, the saliva which bathes the oral cavity, is examined on pp. 68–70, and p. 70 assesses the efficiency of the gingival epithelium both as a barrier to bacteria and as an active participant in the inflammatory response. The mechanisms of the inflammatory and immune responses are described in detail on pp. 71–89 and their importance in host defence against plaque bacteria is considered. The links between these host defence mechanisms are covered on pp. 90–3, showing how they are coordinated by soluble mediators.

5.1 Salivary host defence mechanisms

5.1.1 Introduction

Saliva plays an important role in the prevention of periodontal disease, but its actions are limited to the clinical crowns: those parts of the teeth and gingiva which are exposed to it. These sites are said to be in the salivary domain of host defences, while the gingival crevice and periodontal pockets are in the crevicular domain, because host defence at these sites is mediated by the crevicular fluid and inflammatory cells. The importance of saliva is illustrated if secretion is impaired, as for instance following radiotherapy, when plaque becomes thicker, more tenacious, and difficult to remove. A similar, but more localized, drying occurs on the anterior teeth of patients who breathe through their mouth (see Local secondary factors, pp. 7–9).

Table 5.1   Microorganisms in saliva as a proportion of the total cultivable flora

Organism	Percentage
Streptococcus oralis	20
Streptococcus salivarius	20
Streptococcus sanguis	8
Veillonella sp.	10
Gram-positive rods	15
Gram-negative rods	<2

Note the similarities between this flora and that of early supragingival plaque (pp. 44–6).

A major function of saliva is to act as a vehicle for swallowing bacteria and other debris in the mouth. Bacteria colonize the teeth from the saliva, which contains on average 10^8 bacteria per millilitre, the number falling after eating and then slowly rising again (the main species are listed in Table 5.1). They multiply on the dorsum of the tongue and in plaque and are displaced into the saliva by eating and soft tissue movements. They are then quickly eliminated by swallowing. Approximately half a litre of saliva is secreted and swallowed each day; most of it from the major salivary glands, but with significant amounts of more viscous saliva secreted by the minor glands. Saliva contains a variety of antimicrobial agents including specific antibody and agents such as the peroxidase/thiocyanate system, lysozyme, lactoferrin, and agglutinins. Host defence factors also pass into saliva from the crevicular fluid, although they become very diluted. These agents are relatively ineffective and rather variable in man, but the saliva of some individuals has marked antibacterial activity. The antibacterial actions and constituents of saliva are listed in Table 5.2.

Table 5.2   Antibacterial actions of saliva

A vehicle for swallowing bacteria
Inhibition of attachment of bacteria
Aggregation of bacteria in saliva
Killing of bacteria by the peroxidase system
Killing of bacteria by lysozyme, lactoferrin and other factors

In addition to its antimicrobial activity, saliva, perhaps paradoxically, also contributes to plaque formation. It is a rich culture medium for those micro-organisms which are adapted to live in the mouth, and the initial colonizers of early plaque (see pp. 44–6) attach to the teeth by salivary glycoproteins in pellicle and use glycoproteins, glucose, citrate, urea, and other compounds in saliva as nutrients.

5.1.2 The secretory immune system and salivary IgA

The specific immunological host defences are represented in saliva and on mucosal surfaces by the secretory immune system. Unlike the humoral immune system (see pp. 85–9), the secretory immune system produces IgA antibody in response to antigens on mucosal surfaces. Oral micro-organisms stimulate the system in the gut after being swallowed and the activated lymphocytes then migrate to the salivary glands and secrete IgA (see Fig. 5.1). This passes into the saliva in a special stable dimeric form called secretory IgA (sIgA) and most of it binds to the salivary mucins. The majority of the sIgA in saliva is produced by the parotid glands, although the minor mucous glands secrete smaller amounts at higher concentration. Secretory IgA protects against viruses, toxins, and soluble antigens, as well as oral bacteria.

When sIgA in saliva binds to bacteria their surface properties are changed and they attach less well to teeth and epithelial cells, but better to salivary mucins, and are thus more likely to be swallowed. The attachment of many species of bacteria is inhibited by sIgA, and the effects have been investigated most in relation to *Streptoccocus mutans* and dental caries. IgA inhibits attachment of *S. mutans in vitro*, and prevents dental caries in animal models and possibly also in man. This is achieved by preventing colonization of the mouth and the clearance of unattached bacteria from the saliva. The action of sIgA against existing plaque is hampered because the causative bacteria are already adherent and protected by extracellular matrix. Secretory IgA cannot kill bacteria by opsonization or complement activation because there are few neutrophils and minimal complement activity in saliva.

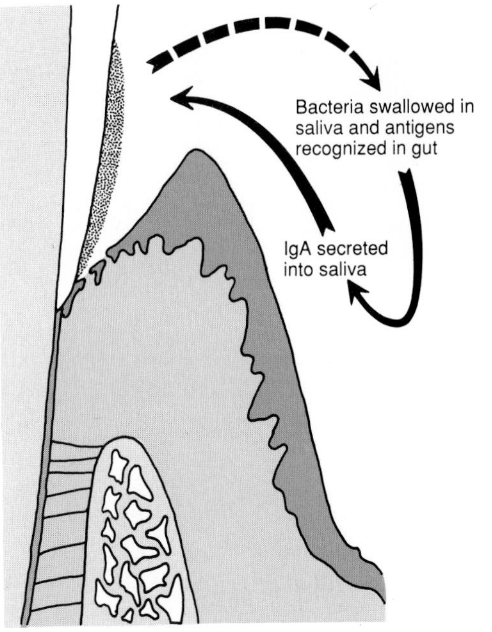

Bacteria swallowed in saliva and antigens recognized in gut

IgA secreted into saliva

Fig. 5.1   Antibody production by the salivary immune system.

5.1.3 The salivary peroxidase system

Saliva contains a non-specific antimicrobial peroxidase system which consists of the salivary enzyme peroxidase, hydrogen peroxide and thiocyanate ions. This system is analogous to the myeloperoxidase system used by neutrophils to kill micro-organisms. Peroxidase is synthesized by the salivary gland acini and

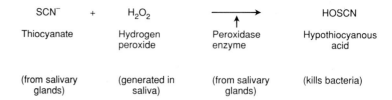

Fig. 5.2   The salivary peroxidase system.

secreted into the saliva, where it becomes bound to bacteria, and thiocyanate is secreted into saliva by the ductal cells. Hydrogen peroxide is continually generated in the mouth at very low concentrations by bacteria, neutrophils, and other host cells, and is used by peroxidase to oxidize the thiocyanate to hypothiocyanous acid which kills the bacteria (see Fig. 5.2). The effectiveness of the salivary peroxidase system is limited *in vivo* by several factors. It requires hydrogen peroxide, which is present only at low concentration, is short-lived and cannot be formed in anaerobic environments or in a low or neutral pH environment. When extra hydrogen peroxide and thiocyanate are added to saliva the efficiency of the system is boosted and toothpastes have been designed to augment this system. However, although the salivary peroxidase system kills bacteria in saliva, it does not appear to inhibit bacteria in plaque or pockets.

5.1.4 Lysozyme, lactoferrin, and other components

Lysozyme is another antimicrobial enzyme in saliva and is secreted mainly by mucous salivary glands with a small contribution secreted into crevicular fluid by neutrophils. Lysozyme degrades mucopeptides in the cell wall of Gram-positive bacteria, weakening the wall and causing lysis. Few oral organisms are susceptible to salivary lysozyme, because their cell wall structure is too complex and because most of the enzyme is bound to salivary mucins and therefore inactive. Although lysozyme may be important for killing some species, it has not been shown to exert any protective effect against plaque.

Lactoferrin is a protein secreted by serous salivary glands which binds iron, an important growth requirement for many micro-organisms. This action is bacteriostatic rather than bacteriocidal, but lactoferrin may also bind to the surfaces of some bacteria and kill them. Saliva contains several other antimicrobial factors including agglutinating factors and a series of histidine-rich polypeptides called histatins which kill some oral bacteria and fungi, but which have not yet been shown to be important in periodontal disease.

5.1.5 Conclusion

Saliva is critically important to prevent the excessive build-up of supragingival plaque and its importance is clearly seen in xerostomia. Its main action is to prevent drying of the teeth and plaque and to act as a vehicle in which bacteria can be swallowed. In addition, saliva contains several antibacterial agents which can prevent bacteria colonizing the mouth and might contribute to protection against periodontal disease. These are effective against bacteria in saliva, but may not provide significant protection against periodontal disease because the causative bacteria are inaccessible within plaque matrix and periodontal pockets.

5.2 The gingival epithelium

5.2.1 Barrier function of epithelium

A major function of the oral mucosa is to prevent bacteria and their products from entering the tissues. This is achieved by epithelial cells which are tightly attached to one another, keratinized to resist trauma in exposed areas, and the presence of a permeability barrier. The most vulnerable point in the oral mucosa occurs at the point of attachment to the teeth by the junctional epithelium, which is only exposed to the oral environment at the depths of the crevice where its epithelial cells desquamate into the mouth (see Chapter 2). In health, the junctional epithelium provides a bacteria-resistant seal around the teeth but, as noted in Chapter 2, it is permeable as a consequence of its adaptation for attachment and is poorly suited to preventing bacterial products diffusing into the tissues. With disease it proliferates to form the pocket lining epithelium, retaining its high permeability and becoming disrupted and ulcerated (see p. 35). Small amounts of soluble bacterial products can probably pass through junctional epithelium in health, and this is even more likely to occur once the junctional epithelium becomes detached from the tooth and ulcerated.

5.2.2 The role of epithelium in inflammation

In addition to the barrier function, epithelium also plays important roles in initiating and maintaining inflammatory and immune reactions. Keratinocytes react to direct damage by secreting a wide range of inflammatory cytokines, particularly interleukin-1 (Il-1) which they release in large quantities from intracellular stores. These cytokines initiate an inflammatory reaction in the underlying connective tissue and induce neutrophil and macrophage emigration (see pp. 91–3 for further discussion on the cytokines and their effects). Cytokines also play a role in cell turnover (see pp. 25–6) and their secretion in inflammation may be responsible, in part, for the hyperplasia of the pocket epithelium seen in periodontitis. Although not present in junctional epithelium, Langerhans cells (see pp. 19–20) are found in the gingival epithelium. These cells recognize antigens which have penetrated into the surface layers of the epithelium and act as antigen presenting cells to induce an immune response.

Because epithelium can induce both inflammatory and immune responses, it is possible that bacteria and their products in plaque can induce gingivitis by damaging the epithelium rather than by diffusing into the connective tissue. Whether the early stages of gingivitis are initiated in this way is not yet known.

5.3 The inflammatory response in periodontal disease

The clinical signs of gingivitis are visible a few days after plaque accumulation (see Chapter 3), but microscopic evidence of inflammation is always present, even in apparent health. Periodontitis is a classical example of chronic inflammation and those features which are not part of the typical inflammatory reaction, such as epithelial detachment, pocket formation, and tooth loss, result from the unique anatomy of the periodontium. It is assumed that destructive periodontal disease cannot occur without accompanying inflammation, because the disease is always preceded by gingivitis and because treatment which eliminates inflammation also arrests disease.

5.3.1 Chronic inflammation

Inflammation is the fundamental response of living tissues to injury and provides a rapid first line of defence against damage and infection. It is non-specific, because the same reactions occur regardless of the cause. This and other features listed in Table 5.3 differentiate inflammatory responses from the immunological mechanisms discussed on pp. 82–9. The functions of the inflammatory response are to dilute or wall-off damaging agents and, if possible, to destroy them. In periodontal disease these functions are carried out by crevicular fluid, which dilutes and washes out plaque products from the periodontal tissues, and by neutrophils and macrophages, which pass into the tissues and crevice to kill bacteria. Unfortunately, although neutrophils and macrophages are capable of destroying small amounts of subgingival plaque, they are unable to remove larger accumulations and supragingival deposits.

Table 5.3 Characteristics of inflammatory and immunological responses

Inflammation
  is rapid;
  is relatively non-specific;
  has soluble effectors: complement, kinins, histamine;
  has cellular effectors: neutrophils, macrophages;
  cytokines are important in its regulation;
  a degree of bystander damage is likely.

Immunity
  develops and adapts to pathogens;
  has memory;
  is highly specific to each individual insult;
  has soluble effectors: antibody;
  has cellular effectors: T lymphocytes, macrophages;
  cytokines are important in its regulation;
  bystander damage generally less than in inflammation.

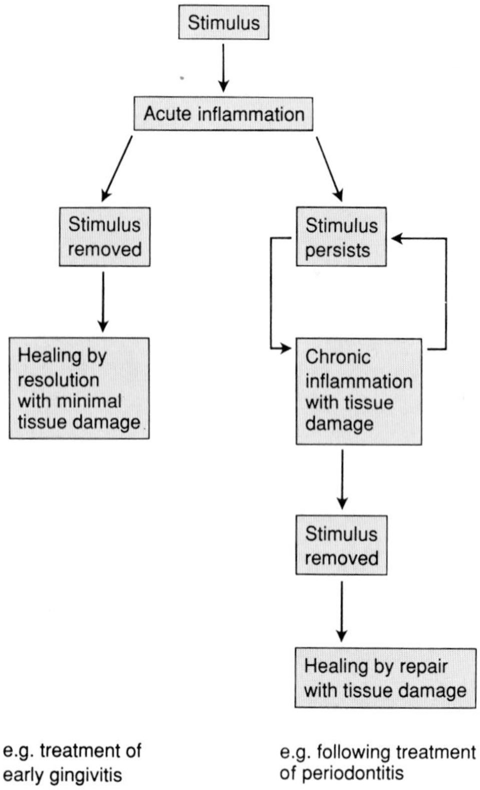

Because microbial plaque cannot be removed completely by the host defences, the inflammatory response in periodontitis is longstanding or chronic. A true acute inflammatory reaction, comprising fluid exudation and neutrophil emigration, occurs in the gingiva only for a short period at the earliest stages of disease (initial gingivitis, see pp. 33–4). The chronic responses of macrophage and lymphocyte emigration become superimposed rapidly but, as in most chronic reactions, fluid exudation, neutrophil emigration and the other acute responses occur throughout the course of the disease. In periodontitis, however, the responses are physically separated to some extent. Chronic responses are confined to the tissues, while the gingival crevice and periodontal pocket experience only the acute responses of fluid exudation and neutrophil emigration.

The longstanding nature of chronic inflammation has important consequences; attempts to heal or repair are frustrated and a degree of tissue damage, so-called bystander damage, is inevitable (see Fig. 5.3).

5.3.2 Inflammation and bystander damage

Because of the enormous diversity of micro-organisms with which the body's defence systems must cope, neutrophils and macrophages have the ability to destroy virtually all biological structures and also, therefore, a great potential

Fig. 5.3 Outcomes of inflammatory reactions.

to cause host damage. In fact, most inflammatory reactions damage the host tissues to some degree. Some of the damage is necessary (for instance the removal of collagen to allow inflammatory cells to function more efficiently), but some results from the accidental or random misdirecting of the host defences. Such tissue damage is often referred to as 'bystander damage' to convey the concept of damage to adjacent 'innocent' cells or tissue components which are not an appropriate target. Each tissue has a limited regenerative ability and can usually withstand the small degree of damage resulting from a short-lived inflammatory response. In chronic inflammation, however, the cumulative damage may become significant.

Bystander damage is a prominent feature of chronic inflammatory diseases such as rheumatoid arthritis, tuberculosis, and emphysema. In each of these conditions the mechanisms of bystander damage vary and result in distinct types of tissue damage, destroying different host components in different ways. Such damage in the periodontium may accrue slowly, as a result of the chronicity of the inflammation, but could also occur in bursts. Unfortunately, bystander damage caused by the inflammatory response cannot be distinguished from damage caused directly by microbial factors and it is therefore not known whether loss of attachment is caused directly by plaque or as a result of bystander damage, but it is likely that both contribute. It is often said that loss of attachment results from upsetting the balance between plaque and the host defences. It is clear that, in reality, there is a more complicated balance between the damage caused by the plaque flora, the protective effects of the host defences, and the degree of bystander damage which results. Although a degree of such damage probably occurs in periodontal disease, it should not be regarded as the major cause of tissue destruction. Bystander damage is minimized by the normal control mechanisms of the inflammatory response and the protective effect of the inflammation is much more important. A small amount of host tissue damage by the inflammatory response is an acceptable price for effective host defence.

5.3.3 Fluid components of the inflammatory response

Inflammatory reactions have two main components, the fluid response, which results in the formation of an inflammatory exudate in the tissues, and the cellular response, in which inflammatory cells emigrate into the tissues. Both fluid and cellular responses, as well as immunological responses, are activated by many components of plaque (see Table 5.4).

Crevicular fluid

The fluid phase of inflammation is generated by blood vessels, particularly the post-capillary venules. In response to a variety of mediators released by mast cells and damaged tissues (see pp. 90–1), blood vessels dilate and the junctions between the endothelial cells are opened, allowing fluid and plasma proteins to pass into the tissues. This inflammatory exudate contains antibacterial agents and substances which mediate subsequent stages of the response.

The increased blood flow and fluid exudation in periodontitis give rise to the redness of the gingiva, the oedema and swelling of the gingival margin, and the flow of crevicular fluid. Fluid exudation is normally limited by the build up of pressure in the tissues, but the gingival tissues are confined on one side only by the junctional epithelium, which is permeable and may be ulcerated, so that the exudate is able to flow out of the tissues and into the crevice or pocket. As a

Table 5.4 Interactions between plaque bacteria and their products and inflammation and immunity. Any stimulus which damages host cells or other tissue components will trigger inflammation, and the resulting inflammation helps activate an immune response against any foreign or antigenic material present. Conversely, humoral immune reactions will often activate an inflammatory reaction at the site where the antibody binds to the antigen

Bacteria and products	Effects
Whole bacteria	Activate complement Activate neutrophils and macrophages directly Are antigenic
Most peptides and proteins secreted by bacteria	Chemotactic for neutrophils and macrophages Are antigenic
Enzymes	Damage host cells Degrade connective tissue matrix Activate and degrade complement Degrade antibody Are antigenic
Lipopolysaccharide	Activates complement Damages some host cells Activates neutrophils and macrophages Is antigenic
Polysaccharide plaque matrix and bacterial capsule	Polyclonal B cell activator Are antigenic
Other toxins, acids, reducing agents and metabolites	Damage host cells Are antigenic

result, there is little increase in pressure in the tissues, and inflammatory mediators which might limit the formation of exudate are lost from the site. Fluid exudation is therefore continuous and it is estimated that 1 ml of this crevicular fluid passes from the gingiva into the mouth each day (see Fig. 5.4).

The inflammatory exudate which flows into the crevice contains many blood components and host defence mediators which may inhibit or kill plaque bacteria, but which can also be degraded by the plaque and used as nutrients. By the time the inflammatory exudate flows out of the crevice and into the mouth it has been considerably altered. Components have been adsorbed on to plaque and degraded, and microbial products have been added. For these reasons crevicular fluid is sometimes referred to as an 'altered transudate' rather than an inflammatory exudate. The continual flow of crevicular fluid has a protective effect, washing non-adherent bacteria and their products out of the crevice and reducing the diffusion of plaque products into the tissues. Flow is generally greater in more advanced disease, reflecting the increased severity of inflammation, the increased volume of inflamed tissue, and the greater surface area of pockets through which the fluid flows. However, fluid flow is very variable, so that some pockets have negligible crevicular fluid flow and may be at greater risk of bacterial products penetrating into the tissues. Crevicular fluid also carries

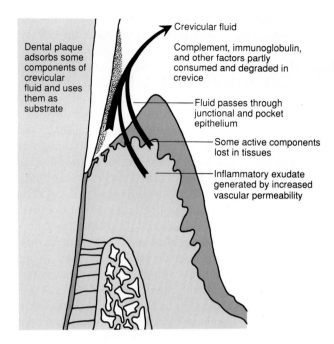

Dental plaque adsorbs some components of crevicular fluid and uses them as substrate

Crevicular fluid

Complement, immunoglobulin, and other factors partly consumed and degraded in crevice

Fluid passes through junctional and pocket epithelium

Some active components lost in tissues

Inflammatory exudate generated by increased vascular permeability

Fig. 5.4 The generation of crevicular fluid.

a steady supply of inflammatory mediators, protease inhibitors which protect the tissues from damage, and host defence agents, such as complement and antibody, into the crevice. The two most important antibacterial agents are specific antibody and complement.

Complement

The complement system comprises nine major complement proteins which circulate in an inactive form and which, like the clotting system, are activated in an enzyme cascade. The effects of complement activation are summarized in Fig. 5.5. It plays an important role in the fluid response of inflammation,

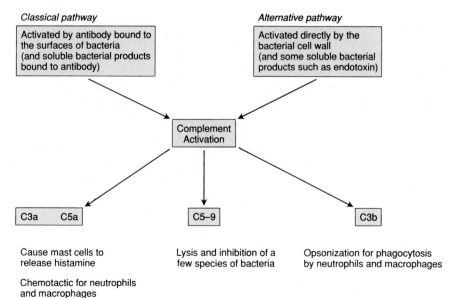

Classical pathway

Activated by antibody bound to the surfaces of bacteria (and soluble bacterial products bound to antibody)

Alternative pathway

Activated directly by the bacterial cell wall (and some soluble bacterial products such as endotoxin)

Complement Activation

C3a   C5a

C5–9

C3b

Cause mast cells to release histamine

Chemotactic for neutrophils and macrophages

Lysis and inhibition of a few species of bacteria

Opsonization for phagocytosis by neutrophils and macrophages

Fig. 5.5 Complement activation by bacteria and its effects.

activating mast cells to release fluid response mediators such as histamine, and it can also lyse some species of bacteria. Complement also activates the cellular response of inflammation. It generates chemotactic factors which attract neutrophils and macrophages to sites of inflammation, and these cells can then remove immune complexes and bacteria which have been coated with complement components.

The central event in complement activation or 'fixation' is the splitting of C3 to form C3b, which becomes attached to the activating stimulus, usually the surface of a micro-organism. Activation can be triggered either by antibody bound to the bacterial surface (the classical pathway) or directly by the bacterial surface (the alternative pathway). Whichever type of activation occurs, a positive feedback loop ensures that large amounts of C3b become fixed to the surface of the micro-organism, which thus becomes a target for neutrophils and macrophages. Antibody may also bind to bacterial surfaces and this coating by complement or antibody, which is termed opsonization, is an important event because it enhances phagocytosis by neutrophils and macrophages. C3 fixed to the bacterial surface also triggers the binding of further complement proteins which assemble themselves into a circular pore in the membrane, a process which can kill some bacteria. The soluble C3a and C5a released during complement activation enhance the inflammatory response by causing histamine release from mast cells and attracting neutrophils and triggering them to secrete prostaglandins, leukotrienes, and enzymes into the tissues. Another complement component, C2-kinin, causes increased blood flow and vascular permeability.

All of the complement components pass from blood into the gingival tissues, crevice, and pocket in the inflammatory exudate, and in addition smaller amounts of some components are synthesized in the gingiva by macrophages. The most important action of complement is probably opsonization and killing of bacteria if they enter the tissues. When there are no bacteria within the tissues the complement is carried into the crevice or pocket in the crevicular fluid, but it is unlikely that it kills many bacteria there. Complement which enters the crevice is mostly wasted, either by being degraded by bacterial enzymes or by being activated by dead plaque bacteria or soluble bacterial factors. Endotoxin, for example, is a powerful activator of complement by the alternative pathway. A proportion of the complement entering the pocket survives to react with plaque bacteria, but many are either resistant to lysis or protected from complement and phagocytosis by a coating of matrix. By the time crevicular fluid flows out of the pocket, all of the complement has been used up.

Complement can mediate bystander damage in inflamed tissues and may do so in the periodontium. When it is activated, a small proportion of the molecules may become fixed to host tissues, lysing host cells and triggering neutrophils to attack them. This is normally a minor reaction, because the complement cascade is controlled by inhibitors in the inflammatory exudate and because host cell membranes contain protective proteins. It is possible, however, that a small part of the tissue damage within the periodontal tissues is mediated by complement, particularly in the junctional or pocket epithelium, because complement leaving the tissues in crevicular fluid would be activated in the epithelium by bacterial products diffusing into the tissues.

5.3.4 The inflammatory cell response

The cellular response in inflammation involves the emigration of neutrophils, macrophages, and lymphocytes from the blood vessels into the tissues. Neutrophils and macrophages perform inflammatory functions which are discussed below, and macrophages and lymphocytes perform immunological functions which are described later, on pp. 80–1. Healthy gingiva contains a few inflammatory cells (see Chapter 2), but a significant cellular response occurs only after the accumulation of plaque (see pp. 33–4). The neutrophils and a few macrophages pass through the gingiva into the crevice or pocket, where they kill plaque bacteria, but they probably survive there for only a few hours before dying or being washed out by crevicular fluid. Most of the macrophages, which live considerably longer in the tissues, remain in the inflammatory infiltrate adjacent to the junctional epithelium. In addition to killing any bacteria which might penetrate the tissues, macrophages regulate many immunological and inflammatory reactions by secreting cytokines, other mediators, and enzymes.

Studies have been performed on the neutrophils in the crevice or pocket using the technique known as crevicular washing, in which a small volume of saline is instilled gently into the crevice using a pipette and the cells are washed out and collected. The number of neutrophils present in such washings is proportional to the degree of inflammation present and the pocket depth, reflecting the surface area of the tissues through which neutrophils can emigrate.

Emigration and chemotaxis

Leucocytes normally travel along the centre of the lumen of blood vessels, but in inflamed tissues the blood flow is slowed by fluid exudation and they adhere more readily to endothelial cells. Inflammatory cells can, therefore, contact and attach to the inside of vessel walls and emigrate out into the tissues by passing between the endothelial cell junctions. The cells move to the site of inflammation

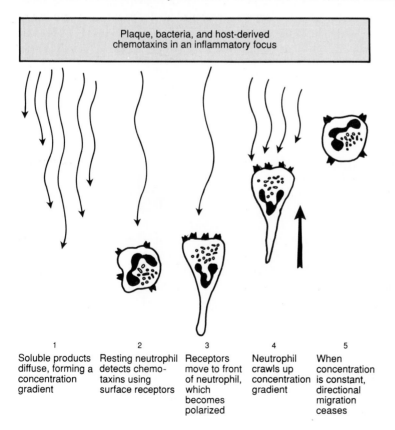

Plaque, bacteria, and host-derived chemotaxins in an inflammatory focus

1	2	3	4	5
Soluble products diffuse, forming a concentration gradient	Resting neutrophil detects chemotaxins using surface receptors	Receptors move to front of neutrophil, which becomes polarized	Neutrophil crawls up concentration gradient	When concentration is constant, directional migration ceases

Fig. 5.6 Stages in neutrophil chemotaxis.

in the tissues by chemotaxis, a process of cellular locomotion directed by a gradient of soluble chemical messengers (see Fig. 5.6). The messengers are known as chemotaxins and include compounds such as complement fragments (including C5a), leukotriene B4 (secreted by mast cells, neutrophils, and macrophages), bacterial products (including lipopolysaccharide and small peptides), and factors released by damaged tissues. Several such chemotaxins are generated in inflamed tissue and many are produced by the plaque flora.

Functions of neutrophils in the gingiva, crevice, and pocket

The functions of neutrophils are well understood from their important role in other infections. After migrating through the tissues to the site of infection, neutrophils recognize and bind to invading micro-organisms using receptors on their surface. They can recognize micro-organisms directly by binding to their cell wall, but the process is much more effective if opsonins, such as complement (see pp. 75–6) and specific antibody (see pp. 83–5), are bound to the bacterium. The receptors trigger the neutrophil to ingest or phagocytose the bacterium into a vacuole within the cell and activate the neutrophil's killing mechanisms (see Fig. 5.7). These include the secretion of hydrogen peroxide and hypochlorous acid into the vacuole and the release of various antimicrobial proteins stored in

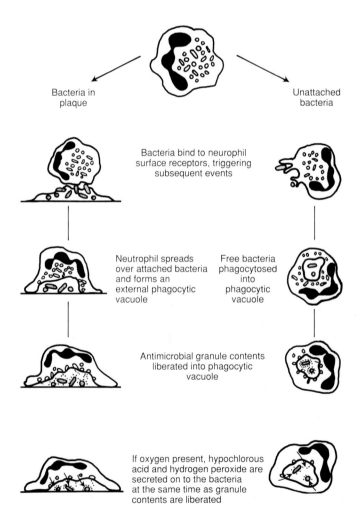

Bacteria in
plaque

Unattached
bacteria

Bacteria bind to neurophil
surface receptors, triggering
subsequent events

Neutrophil spreads
over attached bacteria
and forms an
external phagocytic
vacuole

Free bacteria
phagocytosed
into
phagocytic
vacuole

Antimicrobial granule contents
liberated into phagocytic
vacuole

If oxygen present, hypochlorous
acid and hydrogen peroxide are
secreted on to the bacteria
at the same time as granule
contents are liberated

Fig. 5.7 How neutrophils kill bacteria.

Table 5.5   Antibacterial agents produced by neutrophils

Active only in presence of oxygen (aerobic conditions)
  Hypochlorous acid
  Hydrogen peroxide
  Chloramines

Active under anaerobic and aerobic conditions
  Lysozyme
  Bactericidal permeability increasing protein
  Cationic antimicrobial proteins
  Defensins
  Lactoferrin
  Cathepsin G
  Elastase and other degradative enzymes
  Acid

neutrophil granules (see Table 5.5). After it has been killed, the micro-organism is digested by enzymes which are also released from the granules, and the remnants of the micro-organism are expelled from the cell by reverse endocytosis. Neutrophils can phagocytose and kill many micro-organisms at once, although bacteria vary considerably in their susceptibility to opsonization and to the various killing mechanisms.

Plaque micro-organisms do not normally enter the tissues so, in order to kill them, neutrophils must leave the tissues and enter the gingival crevice or periodontal pocket. Neutrophils in the crevice form a layer on the surface of the plaque, but cannot phagocytose the adherent bacteria which are embedded in plaque matrix. They therefore secrete their enzymes, hydrogen peroxide, and hypochlorous acid externally, killing bacteria without phagocytosis (see Fig. 5.7). This mechanism also solubilizes the plaque matrix, so that the plaque and bacteria can be washed from the crevice by crevicular fluid. Both unopsonized and opsonized bacteria are susceptible to these mechanisms, but opsonization enhances their efficiency. Bacteria which are not embedded in matrix, such as those in the unattached plaque at the depths of the pocket, could be phagocytosed and killed in the traditional manner, but this is unusual. Neutrophils are inhibited by microbial factors such as endotoxins, formyl peptides, and toxins, and by host factors such as degraded antibody, complement, and protease inhibitors in the crevicular fluid which inhibit phagocytosis by blocking the cell's surface receptors. The low oxygen concentration and redox potential (see p. 51) in deep pockets also inhibit neutrophil function (see Table 5.5).

Neutrophils are crucial in the host defence against periodontal disease. When neutrophil counts are lowered in animals, periodontal health deteriorates rapidly and acute infection occurs at the gingival margin. Similar, though less marked, effects are seen in patients suffering agranulocytosis as a result of drug reactions. Defects in individual neutrophil functions, including chemotaxis and bacterial killing, are also found in rare genetic diseases which, along with their other signs and symptoms, all share an increased susceptibility to destructive periodontal disease (see Table 5.6).

Because neutrophils are essential for periodontal health, it has been suggested that the progression of adult periodontitis might be caused by subtle systemic neutrophil defects or temporarily impaired function, but there is, as yet, no good evidence to support this view. It remains a possibility that impairment of neutrophil function in pockets or tissues by the subgingival flora could lead to

Table 5.6   Neutrophil defects associated with periodontal destruction

Reduced numbers of neutrophils:
  Drug-induced neutropaenia
  Experimental neutropaenia in animals
  Agranulocytosis
  Cyclic neutropaenia

Defective neutrophil function:
  Leucocyte adhesion deficiency
  Lazy leucocyte syndrome
  Papillon–Lefèvre syndrome
  Chediak–Higashi syndrome

Impaired neutrophil function may contribute to periodontitis in:
  Diabetes
  Down's syndrome

disease progression at individual sites. Neutrophil defects are much more strongly associated with juvenile periodontitis. A variety of genetic defects in neutrophil surface receptors, chemotaxis, and intracellular signalling are present in a proportion of these patients. The defects appear to be mild because no other sites, except the middle ear in a few patients, are susceptible to infection (see pp. 111–17).

Although neutrophils are essential for host defence, they can also cause bystander damage, and some tissue damage is probably an unavoidable consequence of neutrophil activation. When neutrophils phagocytose and kill bacteria in intracellular vacuoles, the toxic agents and granule enzymes are safely separated from the surrounding host tissues. If, as in the crevice, they are deliberately secreted extracellularly or if small amounts are spilt into the tissues during phagocytosis, they are rapidly inactivated by specific inhibitors in the inflammatory exudate. However, these agents may damage the host if the protective inhibitors are degraded or saturated. The junctional epithelium is particularly at risk of such damage because neutrophils secrete their granule enzymes and toxins on to the bacteria which adhere to it, damaging the epithelial cell underneath.

Functions of macrophages in the gingiva, crevice, and pocket

Macrophages develop from blood monocytes, which emigrate into the tissues from the blood and are triggered to develop into the mature macrophages by cytokines, other inflammatory mediators, and bacterial products, such as endotoxin, in inflammatory foci. Macrophages modulate the fluid and cellular phases of inflammation, phagocytose and kill bacteria, remove damaged host tissues during inflammation, and also trap and present antigens to lymphocytes for the induction of immune responses. Because these functions unite inflammation and immunity, the macrophage plays an extremely important role in all bacterial infections. The possible functions of macrophages in periodontal disease are summarized in Fig. 5.8.

Macrophages emigrate into the tissues in periodontitis and a number continue into the gingival crevice, where, like neutrophils, they kill plaque bacteria. However, many remain in the inflamed gingival tissues where they carry out the functions described above. Many of these are accomplished through the secretion of inflammatory mediators, including cytokines, prostaglandins, leu-

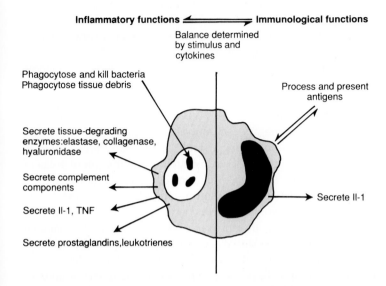

Inflammatory functions ⇌ Immunological functions

Balance determined
by stimulus and
cytokines

Phagocytose and kill bacteria
Phagocytose tissue debris

Process and present
antigens

Secrete tissue-degrading
enzymes:elastase, collagenase,
hyaluronidase

Secrete complement
components

Secrete Il-1, TNF

Secrete Il-1

Secrete prostaglandins,leukotrienes

Fig. 5.8 Functions of macrophages in periodontal disease.

kotrienes, and complement components. Particularly important is the secretion of cytokines and, although many cell types, including fibroblasts, endothelial cells, and keratinocytes, also secrete cytokines, macrophages secrete the greatest quantities. The most significant cytokine in inflammation is Il-1 which is a key mediator both in inflammation and immunity induced by bacteria. Macrophages are stimulated to produce Il-1 by phagocytosis of bacteria, soluble bacterial products, including endotoxin, and by other inflammatory mediators such as the interferons. Il-1 increases inflammation by releasing histamine from mast cells, attracting neutrophils and more macrophages into the tissues, and by causing many other cells to release prostaglandins. It is also required for macrophages to induce an efficient immune response to antigen. Tumour necrosis factor (TNF) is also secreted by macrophages and has similar inflammatory actions to Il-1. The effects of Il-1 and TNF are discussed in more detail on pp. 91–3.

Macrophages, like neutrophils, are essential for effective host defence, but can mediate a small amount of bystander damage. Tissue damage could be caused directly, by secreting enzymes and toxins in a similar manner to neutrophils (see pp. 78–80), and indirectly, by secretion of cytokines. In excess, Il-1 has several damaging effects including stimulation of bone resorption and tissue fibrosis. Many of these effects, including bone resorption, are shared by TNF, which is also secreted by macrophages (see pp. 105–6).

5.3.5 Other types of cell in inflammation

The cells of the periodontium are not passive when the tissues become inflamed, but perform regulatory roles in inflammation and healing, and have the capacity to initiate and amplify host tissue damage. Although they are not primarily regarded as inflammatory cells, endothelial cells, fibroblasts, and epithelial cells are essential for an effective inflammatory response in the periodontium. The active participation of the endothelial cells is essential for all inflammatory cells to emigrate into the tissues. They respond to cytokines, including Il-1 and TNF, and leukotrienes and bacterial endotoxin, becoming more adhesive for neutrophils, macrophages, and lymphocytes. This permits these cells to attach to the blood vessel wall and pass through the cell junctions. Endothelial cells also control blood clotting, fibrinolysis, and platelet reactivity in inflamed tissues. These functions are performed through the secretion of various cytokines, including Il-1 and TNF, prostaglandins, and leukotrienes.

Fibroblasts are recruited to the inflammatory reponse to perform different functions at different stages. In early inflammation, collagen and ground substance are removed from tissues to allow inflammatory cells to move easily through the tissues. Later in healing, collagen is laid down to repair the tissues. Fibroblasts proliferate in inflammatory foci and are chemotactically attracted to damaged tissue by fragments of collagen and ground substances such as fibronectin, and then stimulated to lay down collagen at the margin of areas of active inflammation. These processes are orchestrated by mediators including complement, prostaglandins, leukotrienes, and a complex array of cytokines. Fibroblasts themselves secrete prostaglandins and a range of cytokines, including Il-1, as well as collagenase, collagen, and ground substances, and a balance exists in inflammation between the signals stimulating tissue breakdown and tissue repair. In periodontal disease the balance in the area occupied by the inflammatory infiltrate favours collagen loss, while at the periphery it favours fibrosis. The functions of fibroblasts in turnover and repair are also considered further on pp. 26–8, 105–7, and 134–7.

The important roles of epithelial cells in inflammation and immunity have already been discussed on p. 71.

5.3.6 The inflammatory response – conclusions

Periodontitis is a typical chronic inflammatory reaction in which fluid and cellular responses occur together. The production of the inflammatory exudate results in gingival oedema and the flow of crevicular fluid, and neutrophils and macrophages emigrate into the tissues and crevice or pocket.

Neutrophils are essential for effective host defence against plaque. They emigrate through the gingiva into the crevice where they wall-off plaque, secrete enzymes and other toxins onto it, and phagocytose and kill plaque bacteria. Macrophages are present in smaller numbers and carry out similar functions, but perform other important roles because they control inflammatory processes, secrete cytokines, and are necessary for an efficient immunological response to plaque.

Neutrophils, macrophages, and tissue cells, including keratinocytes and fibroblasts, all perform roles in the inflammatory reaction through the secretion and response to inflammatory mediators and cytokines.

5.4 The immunological response in periodontal disease

The inflammatory defence mechanisms are described as non-specific, because any type of inflammatory stimulus gives rise to essentially similar reactions. The response is rapid and designed to limit the spread of invading bacteria, but an effective host response usually requires an immune response targeted at the specific pathogens present. Such immune responses are more effective because they are self-amplifying and more accurately targeted. Table 5.7 lists some of the evidence to show that immune mechanisms are active in periodontitis.

Table 5.7 Evidence that immunological responses are activated in periodontitis

Lymphocytes and plasma cells are present in the gingiva
Circulating lymphocytes recognize antigens from plaque
Circulating antibody to plaque antigens is present
Antibody levels correlate with disease severity
Antibody levels rise after scaling and root planing
Antibody levels fall slowly after effective treatment

5.4.1 Immunological mechanisms

Immunological mechanisms are stimulus-specific and differentiate between individual pathogenic species and sometimes individual strains. Given time, the response can adapt to changes in pathogens and always has a memory, so that a more rapid response occurs when re-exposed to the same agent. Micro-organisms and their products are recognized as being different from the host because they contain structures which are not found in the human body. These so called antigens (*antibody-gen*erating) are first recognized by lymphocytes, which circulate continuously through the blood, lymphatics, and tissues. Each lymphocyte is capable of recognizing only one foreign antigen and when it comes into contact with that antigen it is triggered to divide several times, so that within a few days there are many more cells with the same specificity. This amplification process is known as clonal expansion, because the daughter lymphocytes are genetic clones of the original lymphocyte and only recognize the same antigen. Clonal expansion gives rise to a larger pool of cells which are differentiated to protect the host either by humoral or cell-mediated mechanisms. Humoral responses are carried out by lymphocytes which differentiate into plasma cells and secrete antibody directed against the original antigen. The effect of antibody binding to antigen depends on the nature of the antigen; if it is an enzyme or toxin then antibody binding may inactivate it. If the antigen is on the surface of a micro-organism, antibody may opsonize the micro-organism for phagocytosis and killing by neutrophils and macrophages, and this effect is much enhanced if the antibody fixes complement at the surface. Neutrophils and macrophages thus mediate immunological defence as well as inflammatory defences. Cell-mediated responses, in contrast, do not require antibody, but depend on clonal expansion to provide large numbers of lymphocytes which destroy targets directly. The secretory immune system in saliva acts slightly differently and has been discussed on pp. 68–70.

Plaque contains many antigens; some are on the surfaces of bacteria and others are soluble bacterial products or components of the plaque matrix, and many trigger inflammation as well (see Table 5.8). In order for these antigens to generate either a humoral or a cell-mediated immune response they probably have to enter the periodontal tissues. Although immune responses in the earliest stages of disease could be induced by Langerhans cells in the gingival epithelium (see p. 19), once a gingival crevice has formed they are much more likely to be generated by small amounts of bacterial antigens diffusing into the tissues. The concentration of such factors in the crevice or pocket is very high, so that a large concentration gradient must be present between these sites and the tissues. Diffusion into the tissues would be slowed only by the junctional epithelium, which is relatively permeable to soluble factors (see pp. 20–1), and the rather variable outflow of crevicular fluid. The absolute amount of bacterial antigens, and therefore also of damaging bacterial factors, which penetrate the tissues is

Table 5.8 Interactions between plaque bacteria and their products and inflammation and immunity. Any stimulus which damages host cells or other tissue components will trigger inflammation, and the resulting inflammation helps activate an immune response against any foreign or antigenic material present. Conversely, humoral immune reactions will often activate an inflammatory reaction at the site where the antibody binds to the antigen

Bacteria and products	Effects
Whole bacteria	Activate complement Activate neutrophils and macrophages directly Are antigenic
Most peptides and proteins secreted by bacteria	Chemotactic for neutrophils and macrophages Are antigenic
Enzymes	Damage host cells Degrade connective tissue matrix Activate and degrade complement Degrade antibody Are antigenic
Lipopolysaccharide	Activates complement Damages some host cells Activates neutrophils and macrophages Is antigenic
Polysaccharide plaque matrix and bacterial capsule	Polyclonal B cell activator Are antigenic
Other toxins, acids, reducing agents, and metabolites	Damage host cells Are antigenic

unknown. Antigens which are secreted or shed from bacteria, either in soluble form or in membrane-bound vesicles, can probably pass through even relatively uninflamed junctional epithelium, albeit in very small quantities. However, the amount entering the tissues rises with disease, reflecting the larger amounts of plaque and easier access to the tissues through the increased surface area of pocket epithelium. Antigens can penetrate more easily and in greater amounts when the junctional epithelium is thinned or ulcerated, as occurs in later disease (see p. 35). These factors are reflected in the fact that more advanced disease is associated with higher antibody titres to plaque bacteria and that these antibody levels fall when disease is treated.

Ulceration of the pocket epithelium would also allow whole bacteria to enter the tissues more easily, and this would trigger an immune response even more effectively. This probably happens only rarely during natural disease, but it may be caused by operative procedures, such as scaling, root planing, or extraction, which damage the junctional epithelium and force bacteria into the tissues. Scaling causes antibody levels against many plaque bacteria to rise and is probably the reason that some antibody levels rise for a short period after treatment. Similarly, when soluble antigens are applied to the crevice in experiments, much higher antibody titres are obtained if the junctional epithelium is disrupted.

5.4.2 Bystander damage in immune reactions, hypersensitivity, and autoimmunity

Just as a small degree of bystander damage is the unavoidable consequence of an inflammatory reaction, so too a small degree of tissue damage accompanies an immune reaction. Any damage caused by the immune response in periodontal disease is probably directly analagous to the bystander damage discussed on pp. 72–3. This is because humoral immune reactions often rely on complement, neutrophils, and macrophages for their antibacterial effects and, as noted previously, a small degree of host damage is inevitable when these systems are activated. However, bystander damage in immune reactions should be minimal in comparison with inflammatory reactions, because they are targeted much more accurately.

When significant tissue damage occurs as a direct effect of an immune reaction directed at a foreign antigen the process is referred to as a hypersensitivity reaction, and several different mechanisms are recognized. It has been suggested that some of the tissue damage in periodontitis might be due to the localized Arthus reaction, a type III hypersensitivity reaction. This reaction can be demonstrated experimentally by immunizing animals to an antigen which is then applied to the gingival crevice. The antigen passes through the junctional epithelium and forms immune complexes with the antibody in the tissues. Such complexes are a potent activating stimulus for neutrophils, which, in the process of eliminating the complexes, cause tissue damage. This constitutes good evidence that soluble antigens are able to penetrate the junctional epithelium and bind with antibody in the gingiva, but immune complexes and the characteristic vasculitis, thrombosis, and tissue necrosis of the localized Arthus reaction are not seen in human periodontal disease. It seems unlikely that this and other types of, hypersensitivity reaction account for significant tissue damage in periodontitis.

Another mechanism by which hypersensitivity reactions can damage the host is the autoimmune reaction, in which the immune system is triggered to attack host tissues directly. There is no evidence that autoimmunity plays any role in the pathogenesis of periodontal disease. It has been noticed that autoantibodies against collagen are found in patients with periodontal disease, but such autoantibodies are found in many diseases and are probably a result rather than the cause of tissue damage in chronic inflammation.

5.4.3 The humoral response to plaque

Activation of the humoral response

Plaque bacteria, their soluble products, such as enzymes and toxins, and extracellular matrix are all antigenic and, as in other bacterial diseases, mainly stimulate a humoral immune response (see Table 5.8). Antigens which pass into the tissues are carried to the local lymph nodes, probably by macrophages, where they are presented to lymphocytes which circulate continually through the nodes and tissues. The lymphocytes which recognize each individual antigen are activated, undergo clonal expansion and differentiate into plasma cells which secrete antibody under the control of helper and suppressor T lymphocytes. Most of the lymphocytes and plasma cells remain in the lymph nodes and secrete antibody into the blood stream. The antibody is predominantly IgG (75 per cent), which can opsonize and activate complement, with much smaller amounts of IgM (7 per cent), which is a more effective activator of complement but a less effective opsonin. These antibodies pass into the gingival inflammatory exudate and then out into the gingival crevice in the crevicular fluid (see Fig. 5.9). There is no primary response followed by a larger secondary response, as is seen in acute infections, because plaque bacteria are present continually. Instead there is a prolonged secondary response of constant antibody secretion, which continues throughout the disease and persists at a lower level even after effective treatment.

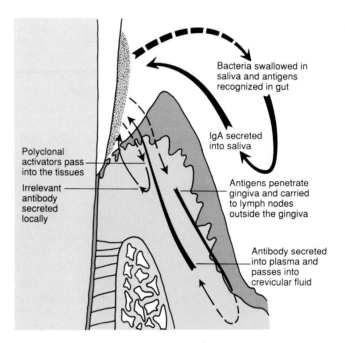

Fig. 5.9   Antibody production by salivary and humoral immune systems and by polyclonal B cell activation.

Although most of the antibody in crevicular fluid is derived from the blood, approximately 15 per cent of the IgG is produced locally by plasma cells in the tissues. As disease progresses and more attachment is lost, plasma cells in the gingiva extend to occupy a larger part of the gingival connective tissue, becoming the predominant cell type in the infiltrate and secreting increasing amounts of antibody locally. Although locally produced antibody accounts for only a small proportion of that secreted against plaque bacteria, its importance should not be underestimated, because it may differ from serum antibody in subclass specificity and target antigens. The plasma cells in the gingiva come from several sources; some are derived from lymphocytes which recognize plaque antigens and have migrated from local lymph nodes or from blood, but many are derived from lymphocytes which emigrate into the gingiva simply because it is inflamed. These latter lymphocytes are unlikely to be a useful part of the immune reponse in periodontitis because they are randomly selected and do not recognize plaque antigens. Lymphocytes which do not recognize plaque antigens should not be triggered to differentiate and secrete antibody in the gingiva, and yet they are.

Randomly selected B lymphocytes can be activated in any inflammatory focus by compounds known as polyclonal B cell activators which trigger them to divide and secrete antibody independently of antigen. Unlike antigens, which only activate specific clones of lymphocytes, a polyclonal B cell activator will activate any lymphocyte and therefore stimulate an antibody response against many unrelated antigens. This is termed a polyclonal response. Polyclonal activation is known to occur in periodontal disease, because plasma cells which secrete antibody to non-plaque antigens, such as *Escherichia coli* or vaccination antigens, can be detected in the gingiva. Many plaque micro-organisms produce and secrete polyclonal B cell activators, although Gram-negative organisms tend to produce more. Examples include cell wall peptidoglycan, lipopolysaccharide, capsular polysaccharide, and extracellular matrix. Thus, much of the 15 per cent of the IgG antibody secreted into the crevicular fluid by plasma cells in the gingiva is probably triggered polyclonally and may be of no value to the host defences. Although the antibody is irrelevant to periodontal antigens, polyclonal activators also stimulate B lymphocytes and plasma cells to secrete very large amounts of cytokines, including Il-1 and TNF. As noted on pp. 91–3 these cytokines can cause host tissue damage by a variety of mechanisms.

The effects of the humoral response

Humoral immune responses are most effective against extracellular bacteria or soluble factors. They are thus suited to protect the host against plaque bacteria and it is generally assumed that they do so, although there is little direct evidence to support this view in human disease. Protection is mediated by antibody binding to antigen and a number of outcomes are possible, depending on the nature of the antigen and the class of antibody (see Table 5.9). Antibody can neutralize or inactivate soluble factors or toxins, such as *A. actinomycetemcomitans* leucotoxin or bacterial proteases, and antibody which binds to important enzymes or structures on the bacterial surface can inhibit bacterial metabolism directly. IgG and IgM antibody which binds to bacteria may fix complement, damaging some bacteria, and opsonize for phagocytosis by neutrophils and macrophages. Soluble bacterial products bound to antibody are taken up and destroyed by neutrophils and macrophages in a similar manner.

Table 5.9 Possible mechanisms of action of antibodies in periodontitis

Binding to bacteria, thus:
    opsonizing for phagocytosis
    activating neutrophil enzyme secretion
    coating bacteria and inhibiting attachment
    activating complement and thus enhancing opsonization
    directly inhibiting bacterial metabolism

Binding to soluble factors, thus:
    neutralizing toxins
    inhibiting enzymes

In order for antibody to function it must gain access to its target. On the rare occasions when bacteria penetrate the tissues this presents no problem but, in order to reach bacteria in plaque, antibody must pass into the pocket in the crevicular fluid. In the pocket or crevice some of the immunoglobulin is digested by proteases, but most resists degradation and a proportion, mostly IgG, becomes bound to the apical plaque. Most is bound non-specifically, but about 20 per cent is bound to antigen and is thus capable of exerting a protective effect in the presence of complement or neutrophils. Such plaque-bound antibody is a particularly potent stimulus for neutrophils to secrete antibacterial agents and enzymes extracellularly on to bacteria and this is probably an important protective mechanism. Salivary IgA is a less effective opsonin and is found only in supragingival plaque, which contains no IgG. Irrelevant antibody produced by polyclonally activated plasma cells is likely to be of no direct value to the host defences.

High levels of circulating antibody are found against several bacterial species, for instance, *P. gingivalis* in adult periodontitis disease, *Prev. intermedia* in ANUG, and *A. actinomycetemcomitans* in juvenile periodontitis, and also against many of their soluble products. Despite these high levels of antibody, the host does not appear to be protected. Instead, it seems that the high levels of antibody are a reflection of the severity of disease, resulting from the greater numbers of these species in plaque or the presence of deep ulcerated pockets which allow plaque antigens to penetrate the tissues more easily. Serum antibody levels also vary following treatment. Raised levels of antibody soon after treatment are the result of scaling and root planing which inoculate bacteria into the tissues, and falling antibody levels long after treatment probably reflect the reduced antigenic challenge presented to the host. Therefore, although antibody levels provide good evidence for the link between certain bacteria and disease, they do not indicate that the bacteria are particularly pathogenic, or that the antibody is protective.

Although antibodies have not yet been shown to be protective in man, they are in experimental animal models of periodontal disease. In gnotobiotic animals, infected with single strains of the possible periodontal pathogens, prior immunization can protect against periodontal destruction. In man, such an association has been observed in the case of *Streptococcus mutans* and dental caries. Serum antibody confers resistance to caries in man and in immunized monkeys, and passive immunization reduces the number of *S. mutans* in plaque. This provides strong evidence that humoral responses have the capacity to protect against oral bacteria, but no such protective effect has yet been demonstrated against periodontal disease in man. Circumstantial evidence has therefore been sought in patients with deficient immunity, but selectively impaired humoral immunity is rare. A variety of deficient and immunosuppressed patients with reduced humoral and cell-mediated responses have been investigated and shown to suffer no worse periodontal destruction than normal patients. They may even have less tissue destruction and inflammation, suggesting that immunity is not critical to host defence (or at least that deficiency may be compensated for by other mechanisms) and that humoral mechanisms might contribute to the inflammation seen in the gingiva.

Depression of immunity in HIV infection provides some insight into the role of humoral responses in periodontal disease, but the findings are difficult to interpret. Patients with HIV infection suffer from all types of periodontal disease, including gingivitis, adult periodontitis, and ANUG, as well as the characteristic HIV-associated gingivitis and periodontitis described in Chapter 7. It is noticeable, however, that despite severe immunosuppression, many HIV infected and AIDS patients do not suffer more severe periodontal destruction than uninfected individuals and only a very small minority suffer from rapidly progressing disease, gross tissue destruction, and necrosis. No simple conclusion can be drawn from this observation concerning the roles of humoral immunity in adult periodontitis because late stage HIV infection is associated with defective macrophages, impaired neutrophil function, the appearance of large numbers of *Candida* sp., and Gram-negative anaerobic bacteria in plaque and, paradoxically, there may be high antibody levels to plaque bacteria as a result of systemic polyclonal activation.

As noted on p. 85, humoral immune mechanisms may be responsible for part of the inflammation and tissue damage found in periodontal disease. In particular, lymphocytes which have been polyclonally activated could be damaging through their excessive secretion of cytokines. As noted previously and on pp. 91–3, in excess these induce bone resorption, collagen degradation, fibroblast proliferation, and prostaglandin secretion, and they attract and activate neutrophils and macrophages.

5.4.4 The cell-mediated response in periodontal disease

Cell-mediated immunity is so called because it involves contact between cytotoxic T cells and the target to be destroyed. Cell-mediated reactions are elicited by, and are effective against, persistent antigens which are resistant to degradation, intracellular pathogens, cells infected with viruses, and tumour cells. Such responses are clearly not suited to protect the host against plaque, which, although persistent, consists of extracellular bacteria and their products and contains the types of antigen which trigger humoral responses more efficiently. Nevertheless, a few cell-mediated reactions may occur in periodontal disease.

The histology of the so called 'early' lesion seen 4–7 days after plaque accumulation (see Chapter 3) and in childhood gingivitis shows proportionally more lymphocytes, including many T cells, than adult periodontitis. This has led to the suggestion that cell-mediated immunity may be important during this stage of the disease. In fact, these features persist into later stages, but are masked by the massive plasma cell response which develops. Many of the lymphocytes in the early lesion are probably immature B lymphocytes and helper and suppressor T cells involved in the humoral rather than cell-mediated responses. Similarly, the fact that athymic T cell-deficient mice suffer severe periodontal destruction does not implicate cell-mediated immunity, because they also have impaired humoral responses. Further evidence that cell-mediated responses play little role in periodontal disease comes from patients with organ transplants, who do not suffer from more advanced disease than the rest of the population despite suppression of their cell-mediated immunity.

5.4.5 The immunological response – conclusions

Many plaque bacteria and their products are antigenic and pass into the tissues where they stimulate a humoral immune response similar to those seen in other bacterial diseases. Antibody is secreted continuously, during disease, by plasma cells in lymph nodes and a smaller number in the gingiva. It passes into the crevicular fluid and a proportion binds specifically to bacteria and their products in plaque. This opsonizes the bacteria for phagocytosis and triggers killing of phagocytosed and extracellular bacteria by neutrophils, and neutralizes bacterial antigens which penetrate into the tissues. However, the mechanism and degree of protection afforded by humoral immunity is not clear. Antibody is probably most important in ensuring that any bacteria which enter the tissues are eliminated rapidly by the action of complement, neutrophils, or macrophages. Cell-mediated immune responses do not appear to play a significant role in periodontal diseases.

5.5 Mediators: the link between inflammation, immunity, and tissue damage

Although inflammatory and immune responses have been discussed separately, plaque elicits simultaneous inflammatory and immunological responses and the mechanisms of the two types of host defences are inextricably linked. The linkages between these processes, which result in an integrated host response, are formed by soluble chemical messengers (see Table 5.10). Their effects extend beyond inflammation and immunity to involve other cell types, such as endothelial cells, fibroblasts, and keratinocytes, so that they are an integral part of a coordinated process of host defence and healing.

Table 5.10   The processes of inflammation and their mediators

Process	Mechanism	Mediators
Inflammation, fluid phase	increased blood flow and vascular permeability	Bradykinin Histamine Prostaglandins C2-kinin
Inflammation, cellular phase	Chemotaxis by neutrophils and macrophages	Complement components C3a, C5a Bacterial proteins
	Activation of neutrophils and macrophages	Leukotrienes Interleukin-1, tumour necrosis factor, and other cytokines Bacteria opsonized by C3b and antibody Bacterial endotoxin

Virtually all inflammatory and immune processes are dependent on these soluble chemical messengers, which form a network which controls tissue homeostasis, inflammation, and immunity. Such mediators have some basic common features: they are generally short-lived, extremely potent, and are subject to rapid inactivation by cells or local and circulating inhibitors. This is necessary because in inflammation they are sometimes generated by positive feedback loops to amplify the inflammatory response and because, in excess, some cause tissue damage. Mediators of rapidly acting responses are usually stored in mast cells in the tissues or generated from inactivate circulating precursors, while mediators of more chronic reactions are continually synthesized and secreted by neutrophils, macrophages and lymphocytes, and other tissue cells.

5.5.1 Mediators of vascular permeability

Chronic inflammation results in dilatation of the gingival blood vessels, increased blood flow and a continual outflow of inflammatory exudate into the tissues. These changes are mediated by a variety of soluble chemical messengers.

Mast cells store histamine and release it into the tissues when triggered by the complement fragments C3a and C5a, Il-1 and other factors derived from endothelium, neutrophils, and lymphocytes. Histamine is extremely important in acute inflammation, causing a rapid, but short-lived, vasodilatation and increased permeability of small vessels. It is probably less important than other mediators in periodontal disease.

Bradykinin is a small peptide which causes a long-lived vasodilatation and increased vascular permeability. It is released from a circulating protein, called kininogen by many stimuli present in inflammation, including proteases, damaged tissue, and endotoxin. Bradykinin is generated in the periodontal tissues and, together with the complement fragment C2–kinin, it probably helps to mediate continued exudation and crevicular fluid flow. Although bradykinin stimulates other cells to secrete prostaglandins, its effects in the gingiva are limited to fluid exudation.

Prostaglandins and leukotrienes are lipid mediators which, unlike the mediators discussed above, are continually synthesized by cells. They are produced from arachidonic acid in the plasma membranes of cells and platelets in inflammatory foci and mediate a prolonged phase of capillary dilatation and endothelial permeability, as well as a variety of other processes. Most of the prostaglandins and leukotrienes are produced by macrophages, neutrophils, and mast cells, but smaller amounts are synthesized by lymphocytes, fibroblasts, keratinocytes, and osteoblasts. Prostaglandins are continually generated in periodontitis and their stable products can be detected in crevicular fluid. Of particular interest in periodontitis is the fact that prostaglandin E2 is a relatively long-lived and potent mediator of bone resorption. Non-steroidal anti-inflammatory drugs which inhibit synthesis of these mediators reduce gingival oedema and redness in man and reduce bone loss in animal models of periodontitis.

Complement has been discussed more fully on pp. 75–6, where it was noted that the complement cascade generates C2–kinin which causes vascular dilatation and increased permeability, and C3a and C5a which cause histamine release by mast cells.

5.5.2 Cytokines and interleukins

Cytokines are soluble proteins secreted by cells, which transmit signals to neighbouring cells to regulate their growth, differentiation, and function. This group of mediators includes the interleukins, which communicate between leucocytes. Cytokines mediate numerous processes, but of particular interest in periodontitis are the cytokines which are important in tissue turnover (see pp. 25–9) and the interleukins, interferons, and colony stimulating factors which mediate immunological and inflammatory processes. These are potent mediators which are secreted in small quantities and act *in vivo* in a complex interconnected network, their different effects interacting to coordinate the host response. Some cytokines are potentially damaging if present in excess, because they can stimulate uncontrolled cell activity, and they are closely regulated by feedback control and rapid inactivation to prevent tissue damage.

It is only recently that cytokines have been characterized, and many of them have previously been known under different names. Factors such as lymphocyte-activating factor and osteoclast-activating factor are now known to be mixtures of cytokines, and all the mediators called lymphokines and interleukins are cytokines. This term is now preferred because many cytokines are secreted by, and act on, cells other than lymphocytes and leucocytes, but their terminology is still rather unsatisfactory. Unfortunately, interleukins are classified arbitrarily by numbers, which give no clue as to their effects.

Interleukin-1 and tumour necrosis factor

Il-1 and TNF are two cytokines which share many actions, and are the most important mediators of chronic inflammation induced by bacteria, bacterial antigens, and endotoxins.

Il-1 is a key mediator in inflammation, immunity, and the organization of healing. It is secreted by a wide variety of cells, including endothelial cells, fibroblasts, keratinocytes, osteoblasts, and neutrophils. However, by far the largest source in inflammation is macrophages, which secrete it in response to inflammatory stimuli such as cell injury, phagocytosis of bacteria, and endotoxin, and also when presenting antigens to lymphocytes. Il-1 increases inflammation in many ways (see Table 5.11). It increases the emigration of inflammatory cells into the tissues and activates neutrophils and monocytes (increasing their motility), anti-bacterial activity, secretion of prostaglandins, and leukotrienes. Il-1 also induces proliferation of keratinocytes, fibroblasts, and endothelial cells, and induces collagen synthesis by fibroblasts. One of the reasons for its diverse effects is that it triggers cells to secrete further mediators. Il-1 also amplifies immune responses and is essential for antigen presentation and an effective immune response. All these effects are clearly important in normal host defences against plaque.

Table 5.11 **The sources of interleukin-1 and tumour necrosis factor and their effects**

Sources

Macrophages
Endothelial cells
Lymphocytes
Fibroblasts
Keratinocytes

Effects
Cause many cell types to secrete prostaglandins
Increase adhesion of leucocytes to blood vessel lining
Cause fibroblast proliferation
Cause endothelial cell proliferation
Activate macrophages for bacterial killing
Activate neutrophils for bacterial killing
Activate B and T lymphocytes for immune response (not TNF)
Cause many cell types to secrete cytokines including Il-1 and TNF
Cause fibroblasts to secrete collagenase
Induce bone resorption

Il-1 can amplify the inflammatory response as a result of all these actions, and this gives it a great potential to increase bystander damage, especially because it can induce its own secretion by some cells in a positive feedback loop (autocrine secretion). As well as increasing bystander damage by neutrophils, macrophages, and lymphocytes, as already discussed (see pp. 72 and 85), Il-1 acts directly on some types of cells. Of particular interest in periodontitis is that Il-1 is a potent inducer of bone resorption and is a component of what was previously described as osteoclast-activating factor. As discussed on pp. 28–9, Il-1 may be a mediator in the control of normal bone turnover and the large amounts produced in inflammation are known to upset bone homeostasis by activating osteoblasts to initiate bone resorption (see pp. 105–6).

TNF is a cytokine distinct from Il-1 and is considered together with Il-1 only because its actions in inflammation are similar. It does not apparently have any role in immune responses. TNF is secreted by macrophages, lymphocytes, and mast cells and increases inflammation by activating neutrophils and macrophages, endothelial cells, and fibroblasts in the same way as Il-1. Some of its effects may be mediated by Il-1, because it is able to induce Il-1 release. TNF can also mediate tissue damage in the same ways as Il-1 and it induces bone resorption by osteoclasts and collagenase secretion by fibroblasts, which it can also kill in high concentrations.

Interleukin-8, interleukin-3, and the colony stimulating factors

These cytokines are considered together here because they all activate phagocytic cells. Il-8 (also known as neutrophil attractant/activating factor, or neutrophil activating peptide-1) is a cytokine secreted by macrophages, lymphocytes, fibroblasts, and endothelial cells when activated by Il-1, TNF, endotoxins, and other inflammatory stimuli. It acts almost exclusively on neutrophils, and is the most potent cytokine activating them for increased chemotaxis, granule enzyme secretion, and toxin production, thus increasing their antibacterial activity. Unlike other cytokines, Il-8 is long acting and resists degradation in the tissues. The colony stimulating factors (CSFs) and the related Il-3 act similarly to Il-8 to make phagocytes more responsive to other stimuli, increase chemotaxis, and enzyme and toxin secretion, and cause the release of further mediators, including prostaglandins, Il-1 and TNF. Because neutrophil and macrophage activation always causes a small amount of tissue damage, Il-8 and the CSFs have the potential to cause bystander damage.

Other cytokines

Interferon γ is a cytokine secreted by T lymphocytes which acts on macrophages. It increases their antibacterial activity and secretion of prostaglandins, complement components, toxins, enzymes, and cytokines, including Il-1 and TNF. Although important for the host response, interferon γ could also, therefore, contribute to bystander damage indirectly.

Interleukin-6 has actions which are similar to and overlap with Il-1 and TNF. It is secreted mainly by macrophages, but also by many other cells, and promotes the immune response. Although it has the potential to mediate bystander damage, it is of interest in periodontitis because, along with other stimuli, it causes polyclonal B cell activation and stimulates keratinocyte proliferation.

5.6 Summary

The ways in which the various host defences act to protect the host against periodontal disease are summarized in Table 5.12.

1. Saliva is important for the removal of bacteria from the mouth and the salivary defence mechanisms are important for preventing colonization of the mouth and attachment of bacteria to the teeth. Plaque levels increase markedly if salivary flow decreases.

2. An intact junctional epithelium is the next level of defence against plaque, and effectively seals the tissues against bacterial invasion in health, but is less effective in disease.

Table 5.12 The roles of the host defences in the prevention of periodontitis. This table lists some of the mechanisms by which the host defences protect against periodontal disease. The first column lists the important stages and processes in the disease, and the second and third columns show the inflammatory and immunological mechanisms which counteract each. The fourth column contains some other protective mechanisms which are important in combating these processes which are not mediated by inflammation or immunity. The last column lists some of the reasons why the host defences alone cannot prevent plaque formation and gingival inflammation

Disease process	Inflammatory protective mechanisms	Immunological protective mechanisms	Other protective mechanisms	Adverse factors which hinder the host defences
Bacteria colonizing mouth		Inhibition of attachment by salivary antibody	Lip seal Washing effect of saliva	Continual transmission of bacteria from environment
Specific pathogens colonizing plaque or pocket	Washing effect of crevicular fluid	Salivary and serum antibody	Population pressure by plaque flora (see pp. 49–52)	Many bacteria are specifically adapted to plaque and colonize the environment despite host defences
Growth and division of bacteria in plaque	Detachment, phagocytosis, and killing of bacteria by neutrophils Solubilization of plaque by neutrophils and macrophages Washing effect of crevicular fluid Complement opsonization	Opsonization by antibody	Oral hygiene measures	Difficulty of antibody and neutrophils working outside the tissues in an environment controlled by the bacteria Degradation of antibody and complement by proteases Inhibition of neutrophils and macrophages in the crevice
Bacterial products diffusing into the tissues	Uptake and destruction by neutrophils and macrophages after binding to antibody	Neutralizing and opsonizing antibody	Outflow of crevicular fluid Epithelial barrier	Crevicular fluid flow is very variable Junctional and pocket epithelium becomes ulcerated High concentrations of bacterial factors present
Bacteria entering tissues	Killing by complement, neutrophils, and macrophages	Opsonization by antibody	Epithelial barrier Obligate anaerobes killed by oxygen in tissues	Ulceration of junctional epithelium Tooth and tissue movement Some bacteria may be adapted to live in tissues
Bystander tissue damage	Minimized by close feedback control of all inflammatory mechanisms, especially neutrophils, macrophages, and complement Minimized by rapid inactivation of mediators Minimized by protease inhibitors in exudate	Minimized by accurate immunological targeting of host responses		Chronic inflammation always causes a minor degree of tissue damage, and plaque continually activates inflammation and immunity Cytokines may be damaging in excess Polyclonally activated B cells secrete large amonts of cytokines
Tissue repair and healing	Removal of damaged tissue by macrophages Recruitment of tissue cells for healing and stimulation to divide by cytokines			Continued presence of plaque

3. Junctional epithelium is permeable, allowing bacterial products to diffuse into the tissues and neutrophils and crevicular fluid to pass out into the crevice.

4. Plaque activates both inflammatory and immune host defences, and both are active together in an integrated host response. In a chronic reaction such as periodontal disease it is not possible to say whether the host defences are activated primarily by inflammatory or immunological mechanisms.

5. Periodontal disease is a good example of a chronic inflammatory response, which becomes longstanding because its cause persists.

6. Plaque can initiate inflammation by damaging the junctional epithelium or the gingival connective tissue.

7. Inflammation results in oedema, crevicular fluid flow, and accumulation of neutrophils and macrophages.

8. Neutrophils are critical to prevent progression of periodontal disease and bacterial penetration of the tissues. They migrate into the crevice and periodontal pocket and secrete antibacterial agents on to the surface of plaque.

9. Macrophages in the tissues control inflammation and present antigens to the immune system. They also migrate into the crevice or pocket where they perform similar functions to neutrophils. Macrophages are an important source of cytokines in inflamed tissue.

10. Plaque antigens can diffuse through the junctional epithelium or enter the tissues through ulcers when crevicular fluid flow is reduced, and these activate a mainly humoral immune response.

11. Antibody secreted by plasma cells in lymph nodes passes from the circulation into the tissues in the inflammatory infiltrate and, together with a smaller amount of locally produced antibody, passes into the crevicular fluid. Antibody levels against some bacteria correlate with severity and vary with treatment.

12. Humoral immune responses, together with complement and neutrophils, are important for the rapid elimination of bacteria and soluble bacterial products which enter the tissues.

13. Antibody also opsonizes bacteria in plaque, but the importance of this reaction in protection against periodontal disease is unclear.

14. Cell-mediated immune responses appear to play little role in periodontal disease.

15. Host defences and the cells of the periodontium are all linked by a complex network of soluble mediators and cytokines which coordinate tissue turnover, inflammatory processes, and the immune response. These are essential for effective host responses but, in excess, some, particularly Il-1, TNF, and prostaglandins, mediate tissue damage.

16. Overall, the host defences are extremely successful in preventing infection around the teeth, a potential weak point in the epithelial covering of the body. They are also successful in preventing destructive periodontal disease

in the majority of the population despite the difficulty of dealing with a large mass of bacteria outside the body.

17. The price of successful host defence is a small degree of tissue damage, caused in part by bacteria and their products and in part by the inflammatory and immunological responses which they elicit. This is acceptable considering the effectiveness of the host defences in preventing overt infection at the gingival margin.

5.7 Further reading

Salivary defence mechanisms

Challacombe, S. (1991). Oral diseases in *Clinical Immunology* (eds J. Brostoff, G. Scadding, D. Male, and I. Roitt). (Gower, London).
— *Includes an up to date review of the salivary immune system.*

General sources of reference for inflammation and immunological mechanisms

Taussig, M. (1984) *Processes in pathology and microbiology.* (2nd edn). (Blackwell, Oxford).
— *Covers inflammation and immunity, but without up to date information on the role of cytokines.*

Roitt, I., Brostoff, J., and Male, D. (1985) *Immunology* (2nd edn). (Gower, London).
— *A clear textbook of immunology which includes the roles of cytokines and some information on inflammation.*

Gallin, J., Goldstein, I, and Snyderman, R (1988). *Inflammation, basic principles and clinical correlates.* (Raven Press, New York).
— *A large and comprehensive textbook suitable for detailed reference to all aspects of inflammation, but probably only found in larger libraries*

The host defences in periodontal disease

Genco, R. and Slots, J. (1984). Host responses in periodontal disease. *J. Dent. Res.* **63**, 441–51.
— *A review paper covering complement, phagocytosis, and immune responses, and their interactions with plaque bacteria.*

Listgarten, M. (1986). Pathogenesis of periodontitis. *J. Clin. Perio.* **13**, 418–35.
— *A review of host defences including a section on bacterial invasion and its relevance.*

Meikle, M., Heath, J., and Reynolds, J. (1986). Advances in understanding cell interactions in tissue resorption. Relevance to the pathogenesis of periodontal diseases and a new hypothesis. *J. Oral. Pathol.* **15**, 239–50.
— *A review of the roles of cytokines, tissue degrading enzymes, and tissue inhibitor of metalloproteinases in periodontal disease. Note that at the time this was written interleukin-1 had not yet been shown to be responsible for most of the bone resorbing activity of the then uncharacterized, lymphokine osteoclast-activating factor.*

Wilton, J.M.A., Johnson, N.W., Curtis, M.A., Gillett, I.R., Carman, R.J., Bampton, J.L.M., *et al.* (1991). Specific antibody responses to subgingival plaque bacteria as aids to the diagnosis and prognosis of destructive periodontitis. *J. Clin. Periodontol.* **18**, 1–15.
— *An extensive review of the relevance of antibody levels to periodontitis.*

Tew, J., Engel, D., and Mangan, D. (1989). Polyclonal B cell activation in periodontitis. *J. Periodont. Res.* **24**, 225–41.

Sutton, R., and Smales, F. (1983). Cross-sectional study of the effects of immunosuppressive drugs on chronic periodontal disease in man. *J. Clin. Periodontol.* **10,** 317–26.

— *A study of disease severity in immunosuppressed patients, primarily with reduced cell-mediated immunity.*

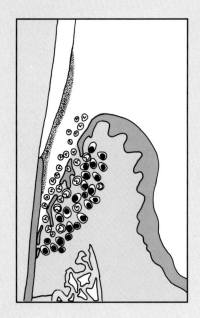

6 Tissue damage and disease progression

This chapter discusses the processes involved in the initiation, continuation, and progression of periodontal disease. It brings together the detailed information in previous chapters to show how bacterial factors and host responses interact in the pathogenesis of adult periodontitis, although the general mechanisms apply to all types of periodontal disease. Specific factors which are important in some other forms of disease, such as localized juvenile periodontitis, are considered in Chapter 7. On this page we describe the initiation of periodontal disease and on pp. 100–2 discuss the mechanisms operating during established disease. The specific mechanisms responsible for periodontal breakdown are considered on pp. 103–7, and, finally, factors which may result in the change from stable to progressive disease are discussed on pp. 107–8. It should be recognized that understanding of these mechanisms is incomplete and the relative importance of different factors is not known in any given instance. There are many different ways in which plaque can cause tissue damage and it may not be possible to predict which are particularly important. However, sufficient information is now available to suggest a unified account of the pathogenic mechanisms which may operate.

6.1 The initiation and early development of disease

6.1.1 The initial lesion

The first signs of inflammation in the gingival tissues are seen between 24 and 48 hours after plaque accumulation begins. During this time the plaque organisms are largely Gram-positive, aerobic, and saccharolytic. Microbial products initiate host responses either because they are able to damage the epithelium or the underlying connective tissue, or because they are recognized by Langerhans cells within the epithelium. Tissue damage causes an inflammatory response due to the release of inflammatory mediators. Neutrophils begin to accumulate in the tissues and migrate into the gingival sulcus in response to chemotactic stimuli released by plaque bacteria and inflammatory mediators. Bacterial factors are antigenic and they initiate immune responses at both sites, which also trigger inflammation.

6.1.2 Early development of the lesion

As the lesion develops, more inflammatory cells are recruited to the area, including lymphocytes and macrophages. Immune responses will result in the production of antibodies by plasma cells and cytokines will be released by T lymphocytes, macrophages, and other cells. Increased fluid exudation leads to an increase in crevicular fluid flow and neutrophils accumulate in the crevice on the surface of the plaque. The gingival tissues become swollen, resulting in a deeper gingival crevice which favours the growth of anaerobic Gram-negative organisms in the plaque. These new organisms produce factors such as endotoxins and proteolytic enzymes which are potentially more damaging than those already present. If the plaque is removed from the tooth at this stage, the inflammatory stimuli are eliminated and the tissues will heal by resolution.

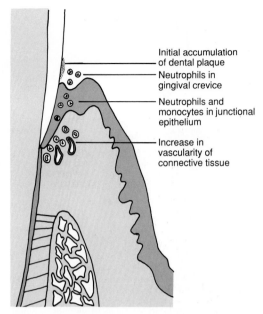

Initial accumulation of dental plaque
Neutrophils in gingival crevice
Neutrophils and monocytes in junctional epithelium
Increase in vascularity of connective tissue

Fig. 6.1 The initial lesion. Features of the initial changes seen in the disease include vasodilation, accumulation of neutrophils in the tissues and the crevice, and increased crevicular fluid flow. Tissue damage is minimal and the infiltrate is confined to the small area immediately subjacent to the epithelium.

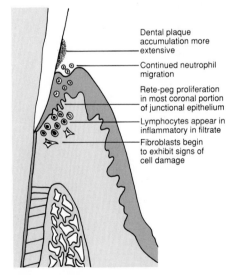

Dental plaque accumulation more extensive
Continued neutrophil migration
Rete-peg proliferation in most coronal portion of junctional epithelium
Lymphocytes appear in inflammatory infiltrate
Fibroblasts begin to exhibit signs of cell damage

Fig. 6.2 The early lesion. As the lesion develops, there is an increase in the size of the inflammatory infiltrate, which contains lymphocytes and macrophages in addition to neutrophils. There is proliferation and rete peg formation in the junctional epithelium, and early loss of gingival collagen is evident.

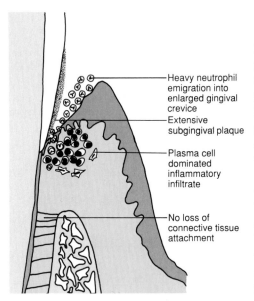

Heavy neutrophil
emigration into
enlarged gingival
crevice

Extensive
subgingival plaque

Plasma cell
dominated
inflammatory
infiltrate

No loss of
connective tissue
attachment

Fig. 6.3 The established lesion. In stable periodontal disease the gingival connective tissue is largely replaced by the chronic inflammatory cell infiltrate and may be surrounded by an area of fibrosis. The junctional (pocket) epithelium shows both rete-peg hyperplasia and ulceration. The pocket contains large numbers of neutrophils together with factors such as complement and antibodies.

6.2 Established periodontal disease

If the plaque persists, the established lesion develops (Fig. 6.3). Host defences prevent bacteria from penetrating into the tissues, but are unable to eliminate the plaque outside the tissues, although they do inhibit its growth. Tissue damage is nevertheless caused by bacterial products and host responses, but is countered by simultaneous attempts at repair. The established lesion is stable and progresses only occasionally, due to bursts of destructive activity which result from an upset in the balance between damage and repair. Following a burst of activity the disease stabilizes and the equilibrium between these mechanisms is restored.

Bacterial products damage the tissues directly but can also act indirectly by triggering host responses. The bacterial factors which cause tissue damage have been described in detail in Chapter 4, and include enzymes which degrade matrix components and factors which injure and kill host cells. The extent to which bacterial products act directly is dependent on their ability to diffuse into the tissues. Although the pocket epithelium is ulcerated and does not provide an effective barrier, their passage into the tissues is slowed by the flow of crevicular fluid, and those substances which do penetrate into the tissues are probably rapidly trapped and neutralized so that their direct effects are minimized. Without these host responses the damage caused by bacterial factors would be extensive and would spread rapidly to the deeper tissues. Due to the actions of host defences the likely concentration of damaging bacterial factors in the tissues is low, but the concentration of host mediators is probably much higher. Host factors which can result in tissue damage are described in Chapter 5, and include cytokines, proteolytic enzymes from neutrophils and macrophages, and activated complement. The normal mechanisms of tissue homeostasis are unable to compensate for the damage caused by the actions of these destructive factors. Inflammatory mediators, such as cytokines and prostaglandins, also stimulate repair mechanisms within the tissues, resulting in the stable lesion described above.

6.2.1 Tissue damage in the epithelium

The normal control mechanisms of cell proliferation and differentiation are disrupted by periodontal disease, resulting in the changes in the epithelium shown in Fig. 6.3. These include rete-peg hyperplasia and ulceration and are the result of a number of mechanisms summarized in Table 6.1. Many bacteria

Table 6.1   Examples of mechanisms which result in epithelial changes

Mechanism	Effects
Bacterial toxins, e.g. endotoxins	Cytotoxic to keratinocytes – disruption of normal epithelial turnover and differentiation
Bacterial enzymes	Damage to keratinocytes
Release of enzymes from neutrophils	Damage to keratinocytes
Complement activation	Cell damage
Production of TNF and interferon γ by activated T lymphocytes	Decreased keratinocyte proliferation
Production of Il-1 by macrophages	Increased keratinocyte proliferation – rete-peg hyperplasia

produce factors which have the potential to damage keratinocytes and might account for ulceration of the pocket epithelium. Bacterial endotoxins are toxic to keratinocytes *in vitro* and other microbial factors have similar actions. Bacterial proteases and other enzymes interfere with the attachments between keratinocytes resulting in epithelial damage. Bacterial products can also damage epithelium indirectly by stimulating complement activation, the release of hydrolytic lysosomal enzymes by neutrophils and cytokine production. Some of the cytokines released during inflammatory and immune reactions, such as interferon γ and tumour necrosis factor (TNF), inhibit epithelial proliferation. Rete peg hyperplasia is the result of increased keratinocyte proliferation and is probably an attempt at repair following epithelial damage. Proliferation can be stimulated by the release of cytokines such as interleukin-1 (Il-1) and transforming growth factor α (TGFα). In addition, ulcer formation results in the loss of contact inhibition between keratinocytes, which also stimulates cell proliferation.

6.2.2 Tissue damage in the connective tissue

The changes which occur in the gingival connective tissue as a result of periodontal disease include damage and death of fibroblasts and loss of collagen and extracellular matrix, together with varying degrees of fibrosis around the periphery of the inflammation. A summary of factors acting on the connective tissue is given in Table 6.2.

Table 6.2 Examples of mechanisms which result in connective tissue changes

Mechanism	Effects
Bacterial toxins, e.g. endotoxins	Toxic to fibroblasts – decrease in collagen production
Bacterial enzymes, e.g. collagenase, hyaluronidase	Degradation of extra-cellular matrix components
Release of enzymes from neutrophils	Degradation of extra-cellular matrix components
Complement activation	Damage to fibroblasts – decrease in collagen production
Production of Il-1 and TNF	Increased secretion of collagenase and proliferation by fibroblasts
Producton of TGFβ and PDGF	Stimulation of fibroblast chemotaxis, proliferation, and matrix synthesis – attempts at repair
Products of tissue damage, e.g. collagen and elastin fragments	Stimulation of fibroblast chemotaxis – attempts at repair

Fibroblast damage

Factors which damage fibroblasts directly are produced by many bacteria, including *P. gingivalis* and *A. actinomycetemcomitans*. Endotoxins reduce cell proliferation and collagen synthesis in fibroblasts, but only when present in very high concentrations. There are many other potent bacterial factors which act on fibroblasts that have not yet been fully characterized. Host-derived factors also cause fibroblast damage by mechanisms similar to those which damage keratinocytes.

Loss of collagen

The amount of collagen in the tissues results from the balance between the rates of synthesis and destruction. Thus a net loss of collagen could result from either a decreased rate of synthesis or an increased rate of breakdown beyond the range of normal homeostasis. Damage to fibroblasts causes a reduction in total collagen synthesis, but loss of collagen also results from increased breakdown by enzymes produced by bacteria and the host. Collagenases are produced by many bacteria, including *P. gingivalis*, *A. actinomycetemcomitans*, and the spirochaete *T. denticola*. Like other soluble bacterial products they may be able to diffuse into the gingiva to act directly on the tissues, but are susceptible to neutralization and degradation once there.

Collagenase of host origin is secreted by gingival fibroblasts, activated macrophages, and neutrophils. Its production by fibroblasts is stimulated by a number of cytokines such as Il-1 and TNF. The activity of collagenase is normally regulated by the presence of the collagenase inhibitor TIMP (see p. 27). There are thus several ways in which the levels of collagenase within the tissues can increase and, unless they are counteracted by inhibitors, collagen breakdown will occur. The level of host-derived collagenase is significantly elevated in periodontal disease, supporting the idea that the damage to connective tissue seen in periodontal disease is partially host-mediated.

Destruction of ground substance

The destruction of ground substance also appears to be the result of both reduced synthesis and increased breakdown. Many bacteria produce enzymes, such as proteases and hyaluronidase, which are able to degrade ground substance. Fibroblasts, macrophages, and neutrophils also produce enzymes which degrade most of the components of the extracellular matrix. These enzymes include gelatinase and stromelysin. Cytokines probably regulate production of these enzymes both in health and disease, with the massive increase in cytokine production seen during inflammation resulting in a net loss of ground substance.

Attempts at connective tissue repair

A number of different repair mechanisms operate within the connective tissues during periodontal disease and these have the effect of minimizing tissue damage. They include the stimulation of proliferation and synthesis of extra-cellular matrix by fibroblasts and are regulated by cytokines and other mediators released during inflammation. New cells are recruited to the inflamed area by chemotactic factors which include cytokines, such as platelet derived growth factor (PDGF) and transforming growth factor β (TGFβ) and products of tissue damage, such as fragments of hydrolysed collagen and elastin. Cell proliferation and matrix synthesis are stimulated by a number of cytokines including Il-1, TGFβ, and PDGF, and by other mediators, such as prostaglandins.

The effects of continuing tissue damage during repair prevents the formation of mature extracellular matrix and the inflamed tissue remains highly vascular and contains only immature collagen fibrils. Although loss of collagen is the most obvious response of the gingival connective tissue to periodontal disease, fibrosis may also occur, especially at sites more distant from inflammation. At these sites tissue damage is reduced and repair mechanisms may result in a net increase in collagen deposition, which has the effect of partially walling off the inflamed area from the surrounding tissues.

6.3 Periodontal breakdown

Periodontal breakdown occurs during short periods which are interspersed with long periods of quiescence. It is important to understand that a stable site may be indistinguishable clinically from a site undergoing periodontal breakdown: both sites are inflamed, will bleed on probing, and may or may not be associated with previous attachment loss. The histological appearance of the advanced lesion (Fig. 6.4) shows the cumulative effect of past destructive episodes rather

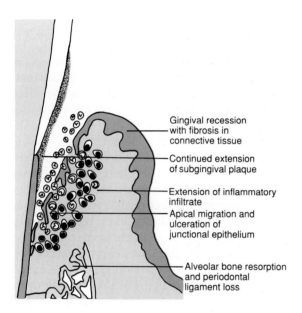

Gingival recession with fibrosis in connective tissue

Continued extension of subgingival plaque

Extension of inflammatory infiltrate

Apical migration and ulceration of junctional epithelium

Alveolar bone resorption and periodontal ligament loss

Fig. 6.4 The advanced lesion. During periodontal breakdown the junctional epithelium migrates apically, periodontal ligament fibres are broken down, and alveolar bone is lost. The advanced lesion shows the effects of past periodontal breakdown and is histologically similar to the established lesion. During active disease osteoclasts are seen on the periosteal and endosteal surfaces of the crestal bone.

Table 6.3   Features of periodontal breakdown

Feature	Possible mechanisms
Apical migration of epithelium	Destruction of underlying connective tissue. Alterations in normal inhibitory mechanisms of epithelial migration Rete-peg hyperplasia along the root
Breakdown of periodontal ligament	Increased host factors causing connective tissue damage of the ligament Increased penetration of bacterial factors into the ligament causing connective tissue damage
Bone resorption	Stimulation of osteoclastic resorption by host-derived factors Stimulation of osteoclastic resorption by bacterial factors

than the appearance of active disease during a burst. During periodontal breakdown, all the features of stable periodontal disease are still evident, but in addition the junctional epithelium migrates apically, marginal periodontal ligament fibres are lost, and there is resorption of bone from the alveolar crest. Ligature studies show that active breakdown may be characterized histologically by the presence of large numbers of osteoclasts in resorption lacunae in the alveolar bone. In these studies a ligature is tied around the gingival margins of the teeth of an experimental animal, bringing about a period of rapid periodontal breakdown lasting a few weeks, after which time the lesion becomes stable again and bone resorption ceases. The migration of junctional epithelium, loss of periodontal ligament, and resorption of crestal bone are closely interrelated and the distances between these structures remain remarkably constant throughout. The possible mechanisms which cause these changes are summarized in Table 6.3.

6.3.1 Apical migration of the junctional epithelium

Whilst much is known about factors which can cause epithelial damage, it is not clear why junctional epithelium migrates apically during periodontal destruction. There are at least three possible explanations for this phenomenon. Firstly, apical migration may occur as a response to destruction of the underlying connective tissue. As the periodontal ligament fibres on the root surface immediately below the epithelium are damaged, there may be a tendency for the epithelium to migrate into the space created on the root surface. Such a reaction is similar to that seen after periodontal surgery, when the epithelium grows back apically until it reaches intact periodontal ligament fibres on the root surface. A second, closely related, explanation is that regulation of epithelium by its underlying connective tissue prevents apical migration, but damage to the connective tissue removes the inhibitory effect of connective tissue on epithelial downgrowth. Finally, keratinocytes are stimulated to proliferate during periodontal disease, resulting in rete-peg proliferation laterally into the gingival connective tissues. This proliferation might also result in the apical downgrowth of junctional epithelium, although there is little evidence to support this idea.

6.3.2 Breakdown of the periodontal ligament

The periodontal ligament
Destruction of the periodontal ligament is associated with loss of the collagen fibres which insert into the alveolar bone and cementum, loss of ground substance, and damage to the fibroblasts. Below the epithelial attachment there is often a zone where partial destruction of the periodontal ligament fibres is evident. The amount of damage is probably determined by the extent to which it is affected by inflammation, which itself may depend on the virulence of plaque or the activity of host responses. The mechanisms of destruction in the periodontal ligament are probably the same as those causing damage in the gingiva, shown in Table 6.2. Thus damage to the ligament is probably not determined by the presence of specific destructive factors, but is dependent on the magnitude of bacterial attack and host response.

Cementum
The main changes that occur to cementum during periodontal breakdown are the loss of the cementoblast layer on its surface and the destruction of the

periodontal ligament fibres which insert into it. Examination of extracted teeth often reveals isolated resorption pits on the cementum, but these are also seen on healthy teeth and their formation is usually followed by repair with new cementum deposition. It is not known whether resorption lacunae are particularly associated with periodontal disease, but they are not sufficiently extensive to suggest they play an important role in periodontal breakdown. It is possible that the factors responsible for the widespread resorption of alveolar bone during breakdown might also stimulate localized resorption of cementum. The loss of the cementoblast layer has not been widely studied, but is probably caused by the same mechanisms that damage gingival and ligament fibroblasts.

6.3.3 Resorption of alveolar bone

The basic mechanisms of bone resorption have been studied extensively and have already been discussed in Chapter 2. In periodontal disease, osteoclastic activity appears to be stimulated locally rather than by the systemic hormones which can affect osteoclast function. Indeed, even where there is generalized increased osteoclastic activity, as in patients suffering from hyperparathyroidism, there is no evidence of increased loss of alveolar bone height. Much of the current knowledge of the regulation of osteoclasts has been derived from laboratory studies, which demonstrate that both host-derived and bacterial factors act locally to stimulate osteoclastic activity by interactions with adjacent osteoblasts. All bone resorption in periodontal disease is mediated by osteoclasts, and bacterial products do not damage bone directly. Like the rest of the skeleton, alveolar bone is remodelled throughout life and, in the absence of disease, resorption of bone by osteoclasts is coupled with deposition of new bone by osteoblasts. Net loss of bone occurs when bone resorption is not accompanied by increased bone deposition. Although loss of crestal bone height appears to be essentially irreversible, the potential for bone repair is not completely lost, and effective treatment can lead to repair of infrabony defects and increased bone density. Alveolar bone is physically remote from the inflammation in the superficial tissues and significant stimulation of bone resorption occurs only during periods of periodontal destruction.

Host-derived bone resorption factors

The main host-derived bone resorbing factors implicated in periodontal disease are cytokines, prostaglandins, and leukotrienes (see Table 6.4). They are secreted by many cells during inflammatory and immune reactions, including macrophages, neutrophils, fibroblasts, endothelial cells, and osteoblasts. None of these mediators is uniquely found in periodontal disease and any inflammatory reaction can result in localized bone resorption.

The role of prostaglandins in alveolar bone loss is supported by numerous experiments using non-steroidal anti-inflammatory drugs such as indomethacin and flurbiprofen, which are powerful inhibitors of prostaglandin synthesis. In short term experiments with experimental animals these drugs reduce, but do not abolish, bone loss during periodontitis. However, in longer term human trials they have not shown a sustained benefit, suggesting that other bone resorption mechanisms may also be important. Prostaglandin E2 (PGE2) is the most potent prostaglandin in causing bone resorption *in vitro*, with the possible exception of prostacyclin. Leukotrienes are potent stimulators of bone resorption and could also be important bone resorbing factors in periodontal disease. Several cytokines produced in inflammation stimulate bone resorption *in vitro*,

Table 6.4   Host-derived bone resorbing agents

Cytokines	Other inflammatory mediators
Interleukin-1	Prostaglandins
Tumour necrosis factor	Leukotrienes
Transforming growth factor β	
Platelet derived growth factor	
Interleukin-6	

including Il-1, TNF, TGFβ, and PDGF. In the past, osteoclast activating factor (OAF) was thought to be an important stimulator of bone resorption, but purification of OAF has shown that it is identical to a mixture of cytokines released during immune reactions, particularly of Il-1 and TNF. Of these, Il-1 is a particularly potent stimulator of bone resorption. TNF also resorbs bone, although it is approximately one hundred times less potent than Il-1 and its likely role in periodontal bone loss is unknown at present. In addition to these cytokines, which stimulate osteoclastic activity, interleukin 6 may stimulate the formation of osteoclasts. The concentrations of PGE2, leukotrienes, and Il-1 in inflamed gingival tissue and crevicular fluid are within the range that can stimulate bone resorption *in vitro*, but this is not to say that these levels are present at the bone surface. Their contribution to alveolar bone loss needs further study *in vivo*.

Bacteria-derived bone resorption factors

Bacterial products cause the release of all the host-derived factors discussed above. In addition, many bacterial factors can stimulate bone resorption *in vitro* and it has been suggested that these agents may contribute directly to bone loss in periodontal disease. Most of the factors are bacterial cell wall components which have been discussed in Chapter 4 and are summarized here in Table 6.5. Capsular material extracted from *A. actinomycetemcomitans* is a particularly potent stimulator of bone resorption. Endotoxins also stimulate resorption at very low concentrations, although they are about one thousand times less potent than capsular material from *A. actinomycetemcomitans*. They may be particularly important because they are released by all Gram-negative organisms and act synergistically with host factors such as prostaglandins and Il-1 to increase their potency. Most of the other bacterial factors are less potent than endotoxins and their importance remains to be established. The concentration of bacterial products near the bone surface is not known, but it is likely to be very low as they would have a long way to diffuse from the pocket without being inactivated,

Table 6.5   Bacteria-derived bone resorbing agents

Capsular material from *A. actinomycetemcomitans*
Lipopolysaccharides
Capsular material from other bacteria
Lipoteichoic acids
Actinomyces resorbing-factor
Peptidoglycan
Muramyl dipeptide
Bacterial lipoprotein

degraded, or removed by the host defences. This suggests that host-derived factors are important mediators of bone resorption, but bacterial factors may also play a role in this process.

Summary of mechanisms of bone resorption

There is good evidence that many potent bone resorbing factors such as PGE2 and Il-1 are produced in the gingival tissues in the course of periodontitis. A number of bacterial factors also stimulate bone resorption *in vitro* although it is not clear if they reach the bone surface *in vivo*. They may act either alone or synergistically with host factors. The host-derived factors which stimulate bone resorption are constantly present in the inflamed gingival lesion yet resorption appears only to be intermittent. The reasons for this are not clear but may be related to the distance of the bone from the gingival crevice, the extent of spread of the inflammatory lesion from the crevice and the effectiveness of host defences in eliminating bacterial factors. As with breakdown of the periodontal ligament, bone loss is probably not the result of the presence of any specific destructive factor, but may be more dependent on the balance between destructive bacterial factors and the level of host response.

6.4 Disease progression

This section discusses some of the factors which may upset the balance between mechanisms of destruction and host responses and which lead to the progression of periodontal disease. These factors are still not understood fully and the conclusions reached here are inevitably speculative.

6.4.1 Bacterial factors

Changes in the microbial flora which could cause disease progression include quantitative changes in the number of bacteria or qualitative changes in plaque composition, and may be associated with direct bacterial invasion of periodontal tissues. Most of the bacteria in subgingival plaque produce factors which cause tissue damage and, as the total number of bacteria in mature plaque increases, the concentration of damaging factors increases proportionately. Thus, simple bacterial growth could trigger periodontal breakdown. The total number of bacteria in the subgingival flora is determined by ecological factors, such as the nature and quantity of nutrients available, and transient environmental changes in the pocket could lead to a short-lived increase in the number of bacteria, increasing tissue damage and resulting in progression of disease.

The presence of certain bacterial species correlates strongly with increased periodontal destruction. Specific organisms or groups of organisms may be responsible for triggering periodontal breakdown. The reasons why particular bacteria are especially virulent may be related to the factors they produce. Many of these, for example endotoxins and collagenases, are common to many bacterial species, but a number of factors have been identified which implicate certain organisms as specific pathogens. For example, *P. gingivalis* produces an unusually powerful proteolytic enzyme and *A. actinomycetemcomitans* produces a leucotoxin which could inhibit neutrophil function. These virulence factors are discussed in more detail in Chapter 4. Periodontal destruction might thus occur when these organisms reach a critical level within the plaque.

Although there is little evidence to show that bacterial invasion of the tissues is an important phenomenon in periodontal disease, it would bring the organisms into closer proximity with the tissues and could be one of the mechanisms that trigger periodontal breakdown. Bacterial invasion would be likely to potentiate the tissue damage seen because of increased concentrations of bacterial products, and would also increase host-mediated damage.

6.4.2 Host factors

As noted above, changes in the microflora could increase inflammation, resulting in increased concentrations of cytokines and other mediators of bystander damage. Conversely, alterations in host responses might result in changes in the subgingival plaque by decreasing the effectiveness of protective mechanisms operating in the crevice. Normal variations in inflammatory and immune function between different patients have been well documented, as have fluctuations in the same individual with time, depending on factors such as diurnal rhythm, general health and nutritional status, systemic infection, and stress. These fluctuations might account for periods of periodontal breakdown, with disease susceptibility being determined by variations in host responses.

In a few cases there is evidence that progression occurs as a result of defects in host responses, which may allow an increase in direct damage by bacteria and their products. In particular, there is evidence suggesting that neutrophils have an important role in protection against periodontal breakdown, including the findings of mild neutrophil defects in patients with localized juvenile and rapidly progressive periodontitis and increased periodontal destruction in patients with systemic conditions which affect neutrophil function. Periodontal breakdown may also be the result of diminished attempts at repair by the tissues, which is seen in patients with impaired collagen synthesis (Table 1.5). Defects in host response and tissue repair may be important in patients who are highly susceptible to periodontal disease, but there is little evidence to show that they are a major aetiological factor in most patients.

Further study is needed to elucidate the full significance of variations in host responses as important factors in periodontal disease. It is not known, for example, if susceptibility may be partly determined by genetic factors (see Chapter 7) and little is known about the importance of variations in inflammatory and immune mechanisms. In most cases it is likely that disease progression results from a number of subtle variations in bacterial and host factors which interact with each other, and it may be difficult to identify specific factors of particular importance in this process.

6.5 Summary

1. Bacterial products can enter the tissues and cause direct damage, but their effects are limited by the effectiveness of host responses.

2. Without these host responses bacteria would invade the tissues, and the resulting damage would be both more extensive and likely to spread to deeper tissues.

3. Some of the tissue damage seen in periodontal disease may be due to the host responses to the plaque.

4. Inflammation results in the disturbance of normal homeostatic mechanisms which control tissue turnover in health.

5. Most of the time periodontal disease is stable, with mechanisms of tissue damage being balanced by host defences and repair.

6. Disease progression probably occurs when the balance between damage and repair is altered. This may come about because of alterations in bacterial or host factors.

7. Bacterial factors which might result in disease progression include an increase in total numbers of bacteria, the presence or overgrowth of specific pathogenic bacteria in the flora, or direct invasion of the tissues by bacteria.

8. Host factors which might result in disease progression include reduced effectiveness of host defences or increased tissue damage in response to microbial changes.

6.6 Further reading

Listgarten, M.A. (1987). Nature of periodontal diseases: pathogenic mechanisms. *J. Periodont. Res.* **22**, 172–8.
— *Review of role of bacterial and host-derived mechanisms in periodontal disease.*

Meikle, M.C., Heath, J.K., and Reynolds, J.J. (1986). Advances in understanding cell interactions in tissue resorption. Relevance to the pathogenesis of periodontal disease and a new hypothesis. *J. Oral. Path.* **15**, 239–50.
— *Review of host-derived mechanisms in connective tissue degradation, and the role played by cytokines in this process.*

Sandholm, L. (1986). Proteases and their inhibitors in chronic inflammatory periodontal disease. *J. Clin. Periodontol.* **13**, 19–26.
— *Review of the types and actions of proteases and their inhibitors in periodontal disease.*

Sterrett, J.D. (1986). The osteoclast in periodontitis. *J. Clin. Periodontol.* **13**, 258–269.
— *Review of bone resorption and the regulation of osteoclasts in periodontal breakdown.*

The factors which are responsible for tissue damage and disease progression are also considered separately in the preceding chapters. Readers are referred to earlier chapters for details of suggested further reading in these areas.

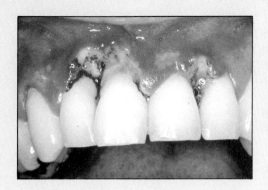

7 Other periodontal diseases

7.1 Introduction

The preceding chapters have discussed the microbiology and pathogenesis of periodontal disease, concentrating on the mechanisms which result in inflammation and loss of attachment in adult periodontitis. Whilst many of these mechanisms appear to be common to all types of periodontal disease, certain periodontal diseases have features which need to be considered separately. In this chapter, the pathogenesis of some clinically distinct periodontal diseases is considered. We begin with a discussion of the features of early onset periodontitis; acute necrotizing ulcerative gingivitis is covered on pp. 117–19, and periodontal disease associated with HIV infection is discussed on pp. 119–20. Finally, on pp. 121–2 the features and aetiology of gingival recession are considered, although this is not a periodontal disease in the true sense.

7.2 Early onset periodontitis

Early onset periodontitis is a term used to describe a group of periodontal conditions characterized by severe periodontal destruction in children and young adults. As discussed in Chapter 1, the susceptibility of patients to destructive periodontal disease varies widely and those suffering from early onset periodontitis appear to represent the most vulnerable group within the population. These patients have been the subject of many studies, partly because of the severity of the conditions in their own right, but also in the hope that they may throw new light on the factors which determinine disease susceptibility in the normal population.

Table 7.1 Classifications and terminology of early onset periodontitis

Preferred term	Principal feature	Alternative terms
Localized juvenile periodontitis (LJP)	Severe attachment loss confined to permanent incisors and 1st molars	Periodontosis (*Historically used term for LJP, not now in general use*) Post juvenile periodontitis (*Term sometimes used to describe LJP when seen in older (20–30 yrs) patients*)
Rapidly progressive periodontitis (RPP)	Generalized attachment loss affecting any permanent teeth	Generalized juvenile periodontitis
Pre-pubertal periodontitis (PP)	Attachment loss in deciduous dentition	

Early onset periodontitis has been divided into localized juvenile periodontitis, rapidly progressive periodontitis, and pre-pubertal periodontitis by Page and Schroeder (see Table 7.1), although other classifications have also been proposed. The term periodontosis used to be used to describe localized juvenile periodontitis, the suffix '-osis' being added because it was thought that the condition was a degenerative condition, although this view has now been discredited. Some workers use the terms 'generalized juvenile periodontitis' to denote early onset disease which affects many of the permanent teeth and 'post juvenile periodontitis' to describe localized juvenile periodontitis in young adults (as opposed to that seen in children and adolescents), but there seems little merit in distinguishing between very similar conditions merely on the age at presentation.

7.2.1 Localized juvenile periodontitis

Localized juvenile periodontitis (LJP) is characterized by severe periodontal breakdown which is restricted to the incisor and first molar teeth. The onset of disease is thought to occur around the time of puberty, although the majority of cases are not detected until patients are at least 15 years old. Affected patients are otherwise healthy. There is progressive loss of periodontal attachment, with the formation of deep pockets, and affected teeth often show marked mobility and drifting (Fig. 7.1). The gingivae do not usually appear inflamed, which may explain why diagnosis is often not made until the disease is well advanced.

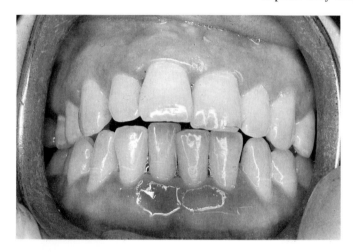 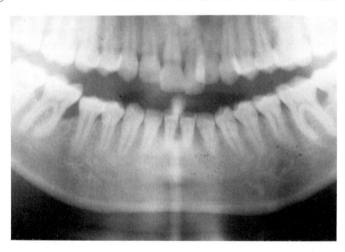

Fig. 7.1   Clinical and radiographic features of localized juvenile periodontitis. Although there is some evidence of drifting of the teeth, the gingiva appears relatively healthy.

Furthermore, only small amounts of plaque may be present. It is not clear why the distribution of affected sites in LJP is so specific, but it is likely that this is associated in some way with the early eruption of the affected teeth.

Epidemiological studies have reported a prevalence of LJP of about 0.1 per cent in Western populations, but the disease is considerably more common in people of Afro-Caribbean descent. The disease also shows a marked familial tendency and some studies have found that females are more commonly affected, with a ratio of around three affected females to one affected male. The observations that LJP tends to occur in families, shows a racial prediliction, and may affect the sexes unevenly, suggests that susceptibility to LJP could be genetically determined. The possible genetic susceptibility to early onset periodontitis is considered further on p. 117. In addition to the severity, distribution of lesions, and possible genetic influences on LJP, there are a number of other characteristics which are distinct from adult periodontitis, including differences in microflora and defects in host response.

The microbial flora in localized juvenile periodontitis

The amount of adherent plaque seen in patients affected by LJP is often small. Characteristically, there is a sparse microflora both supra- and subgingivally, and significant calculus deposits are uncommon. Investigation of the subgingival microflora has shown that, despite the apparent lack of plaque, large numbers of non-adherent and motile Gram-negative anaerobic and micro-aerophilic organisms, including *A. actinomycetemcomitans*, *Capnocytophaga* species, *Eikenella corrodens*, and *Prevotella intermedia* are present. The paucity of plaque is probably a reflection of the fact that these organisms do not form extracellular matrix and are not strongly adherent to the teeth. The flora in LJP differs significantly from that seen in adult periodontitis, with relatively low numbers of *Porphyromonas gingivalis* and spirochaete species, and their absence has been confirmed by studies which demonstrate low serum antibody titres to these organisms.

The most notable finding from investigations of the microflora of LJP has been that high levels of *A. actinomycetemcomitans* are present. Over 90 per cent of patients with LJP have this organism in their subgingival flora, and this is reflected by high circulating antibody titres against this species. In contrast, *A. actinomycetemcomitans* is only rarely isolated from periodontally healthy patients and is not a consistent finding in patients with adult periodontitis. These observations have attracted considerable interest and provide the best evidence to support the concept of a specific organism as a causative agent in periodontal disease (the specific plaque hypothesis, discussed on pp. 57–64). The features of *A. actinomycetemcomitans* have been discussed in Chapter 4. It produces a number of possible virulence factors including a potent endotoxin, capsular material, proteolytic enzymes, and a specific factor known as leucotoxin which is able to impair neutrophil function. In view of the association of LJP with neutrophil defects it has been proposed that leucotoxin is an important virulence factor because it impairs neutrophil function in the periodontium. Only certain strains of *A. actinomycetemcomitans* produce leucotoxin, and some studies have demonstrated an association between these leucotoxic strains and the presence of LJP. However, not all patients with LJP have leucotoxic strains of *A. actinomycetemcomitans* in their subgingival flora, demonstrating that this is not the only important factor in the aetiology of the disease.

Host defects in localized juvenile periodontitis

The idea that a defect in a patient's host response may predispose to LJP provides an attractive explanation for the unusual incidence and severity of this condition. Many patients with LJP have systemic defects in their host defences, with reductions in neutrophil and monocyte chemotaxis being most commonly reported. The causes of this reduced chemotaxis include decreased numbers of cell surface receptors for complement and for chemotactic bacterial peptide (fMLP). Some patients have factors in their serum which block cell movement and a variety of other defects have also been reported. Athough these defects lead to impaired chemotaxis *in vitro* they may also affect other aspects of cell function, such as degranulation, phagocytosis, or microbial killing. These systemic defects may predispose to the establishment of the characteristic microflora seen in these patients. Although it is possible that *A. actinomycetemcomitans* leucotoxin might impair neutrophil function, it is unlikely that the leucotoxin has more than a local effect within the pocket and there does not appear to be one characteristic defect in host defences which is uniquely responsible for LJP. Despite the fact that many patients with LJP appear to have disordered neutrophil function, these defects are mild, as no other sites in the body appear to be at risk of infection apart from in a small number of patients who have an increased incidence of middle ear infection. This contrasts with more severe defects of neutrophil chemotaxis, where repeated severe infections are the rule.

In addition to defects in neutrophils and macrophages, some patients with LJP have poorly formed or hypoplastic cementum ('cementopathia') which may predispose to the disease. As mentioned in Chapter 1, poorly formed cementum also predisposes to rapid periodontal breakdown in patients with hypophosphatasia. The observation of cementopathia in LJP has not been widely reported, but merits further study.

The progression of localized juvenile periodontitis

It is difficult to investigate the progression of LJP without treatment for ethical reasons, but the rate of progression is highly variable (see Table 7.2). In some cases it progresses rapidly to involve other teeth, leading to a severe generalized periodontitis known as rapidly progressive periodontitis. In others the spread of disease is much slower and adult periodontitis may become superimposed on the pre-existing LJP. This results in a clinical picture where incisors and first molars show severe attachment loss, whilst many other teeth may have mild attachment loss with relatively little pocketing. In yet other cases of LJP the disease appears to be self limiting and attachment loss does not spread to other teeth as the patient gets older – a phenomenon known as 'burn out'. There may even be partial resolution of the pre-existing pockets. Relatively little is known about the factors which influence progression of LJP, but the observation that the disease may 'burn out' suggests that age influences LJP in at least some cases. Interestingly, although the condition was once considered to have an extremely poor prognosis, in recent years LJP has been shown to respond well to vigorous treatment including antimicrobial chemotherapy. Successfully treated patients appear very similar to patients who exhibit spontaneous 'burn out' of previous disease.

Table 7.2   The progression of localized juvenile periodontitis

LJP may progress in one of three ways as the patient gets older:	
Rapidly progressive periodontitis	LJP progresses rapidly to cause generalized severe destruction affecting most teeth present
Adult periodontitis	Rapid destruction does not spread to other teeth, which instead are affected by slowly progressive disease characteristic of adult patients
'Burn out'	LJP does not progress to affect other teeth, and the existing periodontal lesions may partially resolve

7.2.2 Rapidly progressive periodontitis

Rapidly progressive periodontitis (RPP) is characterized by severe generalized periodontal breakdown which may affect any of the permanent teeth in patients between the ages of 20 and 35 (Fig. 7.2). The clinical appearance of the periodontal tissues is often unremarkable, although on occasions the gingivae appear fiery red. This appearance has been reported to be associated with periods of active periodontal breakdown, although the evidence for this is inconclusive. The recognition of RPP as a distinct clinical entity is relatively new, and conse-

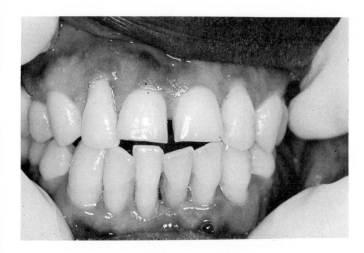 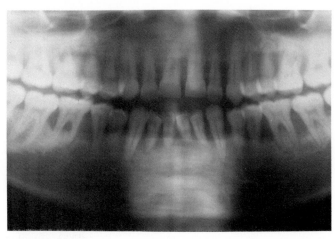

Fig. 7.2   Clinical and radiographic features of rapidly progressive periodontitis in a 23 year old patient.

quently there is a lack of reliable epidemiological data for the condition. However, a prevalence rate of around 1–2 per cent in Western populations has been suggested. There is evidence for a familial tendency and there may be a racial predilection for patients of Afro-Caribbean origin. The condition often appears *de novo* in young adults, although it may also be seen as a sequel to LJP.

The microbial flora in rapidly progressive periodontitis

Although the microbial flora in RPP has not been extensively studied, it appears to have much in common with that found in adult periodontitis. In many cases, plaque accumulation is not marked, but subgingival calculus is usually present in deep pockets. Studies have consistently shown high levels of *P. gingivalis* in the subgingival microflora. Other organisms which occur in a high percentage of patients include *Prev. intermedia* and *Eikenella corrodens*. *A. actinomycetemcomitans* has also been found in some affected patients. These observations suggest that the characteristic floras of LJP and RPP reflect differences in the age of patients rather than being closely linked to the aetiology of the different disease types.

Host defects in rapidly progressive periodontitis

A variety of defects have been reported in host defence mechanisms, notably in chemotactic responses of neutrophils and monocytes. No consistent specific defect has been found in host responses, and it is likely that a number of different defects might result in susceptibility to RPP.

Comparison of localized juvenile periodontitis and rapidly progressive periodontitis

RPP is similar in many ways to LJP, but occurs in a slightly older age group, and in some cases occurs as a sequel to it. The main clinical differences are the age of onset and distribution of lesions. Both conditions often respond well to vigorous periodontal treatment including antimicrobial chemotherapy, but natural 'burn out' of RPP has not been described. Differences in the microflora have been described, but similar defects in host defences have been found in both diseases. Some of the features of RPP and LJP are compared in Table 7.3.

It is not possible to reconcile the various host defects and changes in microbial flora into a unified explanation for the aetiology of early onset periodontitis. It is more likely that there is no single cause, but rather it has a multifactorial

Table 7.3   Comparison of features of localized juvenile periodontitis and rapidly progressive periodontitis

Feature	Localized juvenile periodontitis	Rapidly progressive periodontitis
Prevalence	0.1 per cent	? 1–2 per cent
Racial predilection	More common in Afro-Caribbeans	More common in Afro-Caribbeans
Sex distribution (F:M)	3:1	1:1
Familial tendency	Yes	Yes
Age of onset (yrs)	12–16	20–35
Distribution of lesions	Permanent incisors/1st molars	Any permanent teeth
Neutrophil/macrophage defects	Yes	Yes
Predominant pathogens	*A. actinomycetemcomitans*	Mixed Gram-negative anaerobic

Table 7.4   Proposed aetiological factors in early onset periodontitis

Possible aetiological factor	Comments
Actinobacillus actinomycetemcomitans	Virulent organism which is particularly associated with localized juvenile periodontitis. Produces a leucotoxin which could impair neutrophil function locally
Porphyromonas gingivalis	Organism particularly associated with rapidly progressive periodontitis and adult periodontitis. Produces powerful proteolytic enzyme which may be important in virulence
Systemic neutrophil defects	A variety of mild neutrophil defects are associated with all types of early onset periodontitis. These do not appear to predispose to other infections
Genetic influences	Genetic factors may predispose to early onset periodontitis by affecting host susceptibility. There is little evidence to support the idea of a single gene defect as a cause of disease
Cementopathia	Reports of poorly formed or hypoplastic cementum which might predispose to disease merit further investigation

aetiology, the clinical picture being determined by a number of different factors which vary in importance between one affected patient and the next. Some of these proposed aetiological factors are summarized in Table 7.4.

7.2.3   Pre-pubertal periodontitis

Pre-pubertal periodontitis (PP) is an extremely rare form of periodontal disease, characterized by severe periodontal destruction which affects the deciduous dentition. With the exception of this condition, periodontal disease is not a major problem in the deciduous dentition, although some studies have reported that mild periodontal breakdown of around a millimetre is frequently seen. Both localized and generalized forms of PP have been described according to whether or not all the teeth are affected. In generalized PP, all deciduous teeth show severe periodontal breakdown and the gingivae appear fiery red, and affected patients have frequent middle ear and other bacterial infections. Some reports suggest that generalized PP is one of the presenting signs of of a rare disease known as leucocyte adhesion deficiency, a condition in which neutrophils and monocytes fail to emigrate out of blood vessels because they are unable to adhere to endothelial cells.

Localized pre-pubertal periodontitis is seen in patients who appear to be otherwise healthy and affects only some of the deciduous teeth. The gingiva do not usually appear particularly inflamed or swollen. Few cases have been described and its pathogenesis is unknown, but it appears that the microflora from affected subgingival sites is similar to that seen in LJP, with high levels of *A. actinomycetemcomitans*. Neutrophils and monocytes exhibit chemotactic defects in some patients. There is insufficient evidence to be certain about genetic influences in this condition, although there is evidence for a familial pattern. In general it responds poorly to treatment and may precede LJP and RPP in the permanent dentition.

7.2.4 Genetic influences in early onset periodontitis

The suggestion that localized juvenile, rapidly progressive, and pre-pubertal periodontitis could be due to genetic defects has arisen because these diseases are more common in certain racial groups, may affect females more than males, and occur in families. Families have been described where a number of members are affected by the different forms of early onset periodontitis. It is possible that genetic influences could predispose to periodontal disease in the same way that there are genetic influences in many other diseases. Some research workers have variously suggested that localized juvenile periodontitis might be an autosomal recessive disorder or a sex-linked dominant condition with incomplete penetrance, where not all the subjects who inherit the genes actually develop the disease. However, given the wide variations in microflora, host factors, and clinical presentations, it is unlikely that there is a simple inheritance pattern of early onset periodontitis. These patterns of disease might also be due to environmental factors, such as dietary differences or transmission of pathogenic bacteria between close relatives, rather than genetic factors. There is no convincing evidence that familial and racial variations affect the prevalence of adult periodontitis.

7.3 Acute necrotizing ulcerative periodontitis

7.3.1 Clinical and histological features of ANUG

Acute necrotizing ulcerative gingivitis (ANUG) is a specific destructive periodontal disease characterized by the presence of necrotic ulcers affecting the interdental papillae and which may spread laterally along the gingival margins. The ulcers are painful, covered by a greyish slough and have a characteristic 'punched out' appearance (See Fig. 7.3). Lesions may extend to affect the gingiva around all the teeth, although they are often more localized to the anterior teeth or to one quadrant of the dentition. There are not usually any systemic

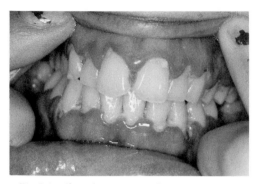

Fig. 7.3 Clinical appearance of acute necrotizing ulcerative gingivitis affecting gingiva around lower incisors.

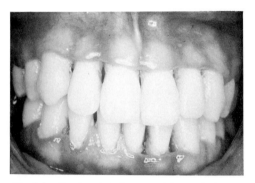

Fig. 7.4 Characteristic features of the residual damage following recurrent ANUG, resulting in interdental cratering and loss of interdental papillae.

symptoms, although slight lymphadenopathy is sometimes present. A characteristic halitosis (foetor oris) is often associated with the condition. The onset of ANUG is acute and, in the absence of treatment, it may last for a couple of weeks, before healing to leave a chronic gingivitis. ANUG tends to recur unless it is treated, resulting in progressive destruction of the periodontal tissues, typically with loss of interdental papillae and formation of 'gingival craters' (see Fig. 7.4).

In Western countries, ANUG is seen almost exclusively in the 16–30 year old age group. Epidemiological studies carried out in the 1950s and 1960s reported an incidence of ANUG of up to 5 per cent in young adults, typically in groups of military recruits or college students. However, the condition appears to have become much less common over the past 15 years, although a similar but more chronic condition may be seen in patients with HIV infection. This possibility should be considered in the differential diagnosis of acute ulcerative gingivitis. The main factors which predispose to ANUG are poor oral hygiene, smoking, and emotional stress. The reduction in the incidence observed over the last decade may reflect improved general health and nutrition and better levels of plaque control.

The histopathological changes seen in ANUG are non-specific. The epithelium and superficial connective tissue contain a dense neutrophil infiltrate, and the ulcers are covered by a slough which contains abundant bacteria. The remaining tissue shows evidence of superficial necrosis, with many bacteria infiltrating the surface layers. The deeper tissues remain viable and are infiltrated by plasma cells and macrophages. The degree of penetration of the tissues by microorganisms is unusual when compared to other periodontal conditions.

7.3.2 Microbiology of ANUG

ANUG is a mixed bacterial infection caused by a group of anaerobic organisms consisting of spirochaetes and fusiform bacteria which is sometimes termed a 'fuso-spirochaetal complex'. These species include spirochaetes such as *T. denticola*, fusiforms such as *F. nucleatum*, and *Prev. intermedia*. The presence of these organisms is supported by the finding of high serum antibody levels to them, and their aetiological role is suggested by the fact that ANUG resolves rapidly following short term treatment with metronidazole, an antibacterial agent which is active against anaerobic organisms. Although ANUG is typically associated with these bacteria, other species, including *Selenomonas* sp., *Veillonella* sp., and *Peptostreptococcus* have been recovered from affected sites. The microflora present in ANUG is qualitatively similar to that isolated from subgingival sites in other periodontal diseases; possible virulence factors associated with these organisms have been described in Chapter 4 and include endotoxins, bacterial enzymes, and other toxins.

There are many reports of outbreaks of ANUG occurring in closely confined groups of young adults, notably amongst soldiers during the First World War when it was termed 'trench mouth'. However there is no evidence that the condition is transmissible. This view is supported by experiments in which the inoculation of micro-organisms from affected to healthy animals did not result in development of ANUG except when the recipients were severely immunosuppressed. It is thought that reported outbreaks of ANUG may reflect common exposure to stressful conditions and poor hygiene, rather than the direct transmission of an infectious agent.

7.3.3 Host response and predisposing factors

It is not clear what triggers the onset of ANUG or why it is normally confined to such a narrow age group. There is no convincing evidence that an altered host response is an important predisposing factor in most cases of the disease. However, as noted earlier, many patients with HIV infection may develop a condition similar to ANUG, and it is possible to induce ANUG in animals following pronounced immunosuppression. Such evidence suggests that suppressed immune function might, on occasions, act as a predisposing factor. Poor oral hygiene, smoking, and stress are strongly associated with ANUG, although the reasons for this are unclear. ANUG usually develops when there are high levels of plaque and pre-existing gingivitis; in the rare cases where it develops in the presence of good oral hygiene it is usually very mild. A number of studies have reported that smoking is an important predisposing factor for ANUG. Those who smoke tend to have poorer oral hygiene than matched controls, but this association is not sufficient to account fully for the strong correlation between smoking and ANUG. Smoking may cause constriction of the gingival blood vessels, predisposing to colonization by anaerobic organisms, and this might explain its mode of action in ANUG. The objective study of the relationship of emotional stress to disease is difficult and there are only a few well-controlled studies which demonstrate the association of stress with ANUG, although the link is well recognized by clinicians. Stress may lead to an alteration in behaviour, such as increasing smoking and decreasing oral hygiene measures, as well as having an effect on salivary flow, the local blood flow, and immune function, although none of these factors appears to explain the relationship fully.

In some developing countries, particularly in Africa, ANUG is seen in children, and is often associated with nutritional deficiencies or diseases such as measles. In these cases the condition may spread from the gingiva to affect the facial tissues, when the condition is known as cancrum oris or noma, and may result in massive oro-facial necrosis. This life-threatening complication of ANUG is not seen in Western countries, although it has some similarities with the severe, but less extensive, tissue necrosis seen in HIV-associated periodontitis (see p. 120).

7.4 HIV-related periodontal disease

Infection with the human immunodeficiency virus (HIV) leads to a reduction in the number of functioning T helper lymphocytes, resulting in the progressive loss of immune function and susceptibility to opportunistic infections seen in AIDS (acquired immune deficiency syndrome). The stages of HIV infection have been classified according to their characteristic features by the Center for Disease Control (CDC) in the United States (see Table 7.5). Periodontal disease can be a

Table 7.5   CDC Classification of patients with HIV infection

Group I	Acute HIV infection
Group II	Asymptomatic HIV infection
Group III	Persistent generalized lymphadenopathy
Group IV	Clinical symptoms of HIV infection, opportunistic infections, neoplasms, neurological disorders

feature of stages II–IV of HIV infection and may be confined to the gingivae, or spread rapidly to affect the underlying periodontal tissues. An increased prevalence of all types of periodontal disease, including gingivitis, adult periodontitis, and rapidly progressive periodontitis is seen in patients with HIV infection. In addition, some patients in the later stages of the infection suffer from the unusual and characteristic HIV-associated gingivitis and periodontitis described here. The prevalence of these conditions in patients with HIV infection is not known, but they appear to be a relatively unusual problem.

7.4.1 HIV-associated gingivitis

HIV-associated gingivitis is a readily recognizable, though uncommon, manifestation of HIV infection. It occurs before other opportunistic infections, and can be an early presenting symptom. It appears as an unusually erythematous generalized marginal gingivitis, affecting a wide band of both the free and attached gingivae and resembles the desquamative gingivitis seen in lichen planus and vesiculo-bullous disorders (Fig. 7.5). Gingival bleeding may be profuse. The aetiology of HIV-associated gingivitis is not yet understood, but it responds poorly to normal plaque control measures. Although the microbiology of HIV-associated gingivitis has not been extensively investigated, there is evidence that the flora is unlike that seen in chronic gingivitis, with large numbers of possible pathogens (including *P. gingivalis*, *A. actinomycetemcomitans*, and *F. nucleatum*) which are more usually associated with subgingival than supragingival plaque being present. In addition, fungi such as *Candida* sp., which are not normally seen in plaque, have been isolated, but their significance is not yet understood.

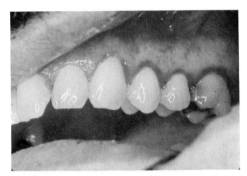

Fig. 7.5 HIV-associated gingivitis. Erythematous band around attached gingiva on posterior teeth.

7.4.2 HIV-associated periodontitis

HIV-associated periodontitis may resemble ANUG and starts with the characteristic painful necrotic ulcers affecting the inter-dental papillae. Although its association with disease severity is not known, it is more often seen in late stages of HIV infection when the ratio of helper to suppressor T lymphocytes is depressed and other opportunistic infections may be apparent. Unlike ANUG in other patients, the condition is persistent and can lead to very rapid destruction of the underlying periodontal support (Fig. 7.6). In severe cases, inflammation and necrosis may affect the whole of the attached gingivae and extend on to the alveolar mucosa, exposing necrotic areas of crestal bone, although pocket formation is not prominent. Affected patients often suffer from deep-seated pain from within the jaws. Teeth may be exfoliated rapidly due to the tissue destruction. The condition usually responds to vigorous antibacterial therapy, including mechanical debridement, removal of necrotic tissue, and antimicrobial chemotherapy with agents such as metronidazole.

The bacterial flora associated with HIV periodontitis does not appear to be substantially different from those seen in ANUG or adult periodontitis. An increase in the proportion of *P. gingivalis*, *Eikenella* and *Wolinella* species has been reported. However, *Candida* species have been found in the subgingival plaque and they may constitute a high percentage of the total flora. Further studies are required to determine the significance of these micro-organisms and of other opportunistic pathogens not usually found in plaque.

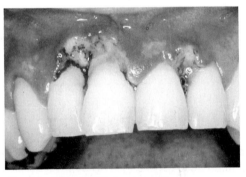

Fig. 7.6 HIV-associated periodontitis.

7.5 Gingival recession

Gingival recession is the apical migration of the gingival margin below the amelo-cemental junction. It is often confined to a single surface of the tooth, typically the labial aspect, and consequently does not usually jeopardize the periodontal support of the tooth. Gingival recession is caused by inflammation or chronic minor trauma if certain predisposing factors are present, or it may follow periodontal treatment (see Table 7.6). In the past there has been some controversy as to whether recession may be a physiological process and a normal part of ageing, but there is little evidence to support this view.

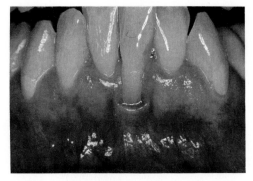

Fig. 7.7 Isolated area of gingival recession induced by periodontal disease.

Table 7.6   The aetiology of gingival recession

Primary cause	Predisposing factors
Periodontal disease resulting in attachment loss	Reduced thickness of overlying bone and gingiva High frenal attachments
Chronic minor trauma – e.g. from toothbrushing	Reduced thickness of overlying bone and gingiva
Periodontal treatment	Reduced thickness of overlying bone and gingiva Extensive prior tissue damage from disease Surgical removal of tissue during treatment

Periodontal disease is an important cause of recession. Plaque accumulation leads to gingivitis and inflammation may spread to the underlying periodontal attachment. Although this normally results in pocket formation, attachment loss may manifest as recession at sites where the gingival tissues are particularly thin (Fig. 7.7). Recession is also seen following chronic minor trauma to the gingiva, such as may occur with regular vigorous scrubbing during tooth-brushing (Fig. 7.8). In these cases, the gingiva does not appear inflamed, but retains its pink healthy appearance. Following periodontal treatment recession is often pronounced, and may not be confined to the areas of the mouth where it is usually seen (Fig. 7.9). This reflects the destruction of tissue that has occurred during the disease process, and the shrinkage of the tissues that occurs during healing. Such recession may be exacerbated by the removal of tissue by surgical procedures.

The principal predisposing factor which determines whether recession occurs at any particular area is the anatomy of the site, specifically the thickness of the alveolar bone and overlying gingiva. Recession is commonly seen labially on the lower incisor teeth and buccally on the upper canine teeth, where the bone is thin, although teeth which are malpositioned out of the line of the arch may also have a reduced thickness of overlying bone and gingivae. In extreme cases, the alveolar bone may be totally absent over the root surface (termed a dehiscence), or a window of bone may be missing (termed a fenestration), so that the root is covered only by gingival soft tissue (Fig. 7.10). In such cases, affected teeth are extremely susceptible to gingival recession. Soft tissue anomalies, such as high frenal attachments, may accelerate gingival recession by preventing adequate plaque removal and possibly also by transmitting movements of the soft tissues to the gingival margin.

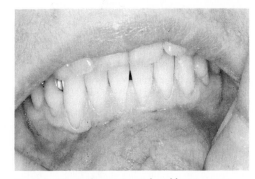

Fig. 7.8 Gingival recession induced by persistent toothbrushing trauma.

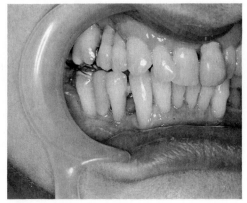

Fig. 7.9 Gingival recession following successful periodontal treatment. The recession is associated with areas of previous tissue damage, and is consequently more widely distributed than recession due to chronic trauma.

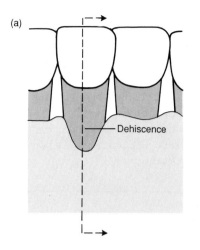

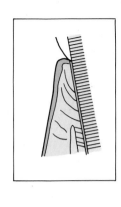

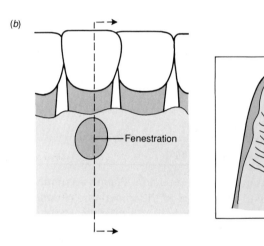

Fig. 7.10 Bony defects predisposing to gingival recession (labial views show alveolar bone defects; cross sectional views show the defects together with the overlying gingiva).

(a) Labial and longitudinal cross sectional view of a bony dehiscence, where alveolar bone is absent over part of the tooth root. Dehiscences are commonly seen where a tooth is slightly proclined, as shown in this diagram.

(b) Labial and longitudinal cross sectional view of a bony fenestration, where a window of alveolar bone is absent over a root surface. The thinness of the bone predisposes to recession. If a small amount of crestal bone is lost, the fenenestration will be converted into a dehiscence.

The pathogenesis of gingival recession is not fully understood, and there are relatively few studies which have addressed this question. Histological studies of experimentally induced gingival recession in animal models have suggested that gingival recession may occur as a result of rete-peg hyperplasia in the epithelium of thin gingiva. The stimulus for rete peg hyperplasia could be plaque-induced inflammation or the chronic minor trauma referred to above, but it is not clear why this may result in gingival recession.

7.6 Summary

7.6.1 Early onset periodontitis

1. Early onset periodontitis can be divided into localized juvenile periodontitis, rapidly progressive periodontitis, and pre-pubertal periodontitis.

2. Many cases are associated with defects in neutrophil and monocyte chemotaxis, or with other minor defects in host defences. These defects do not usually predispose to other more serious systemic diseases.

3. There is often a characteristic microflora, with high levels of *A. actinomycetemcomitans* being found, particularly in cases of localized juvenile periodontitis.

4. Other proposed aetiological factors include defects in cementum formation and genetic factors. There is a familial tendency and racial predilection in the prevalence of early onset periodontitis, but little evidence to support the hypothesis that a single gene defect is responsible for the condition.

7.6.2 Acute necrotizing ulcerative gingivitis

1. ANUG is characterized clinically by the presence of painful necrotic ulcers at the gingival margins, particularly affecting the interdental papillae. It affects young adults almost exclusively and its prevalence appears to have declined sharply in recent years.

2. Predisposing factors for ANUG may include poor oral hygiene, smoking, stress, and immunological deficiency. The mechanisms of action of these factors are not fully understood. Nutritional deficiency may play an important aetiological role in ANUG in some African countries.

3. The microflora associated with ANUG include large numbers of spirochaetes, amongst them *T. denticola*, and anaerobic bacteria such as *Prev. intermedia* and *Fusobacteria*. These bacteria invade the superficial gingival tissues.

4. Although the prevalence of ANUG has declined markedly, an ANUG-like periodontal disease may be seen in patients with HIV infection.

7.6.3 HIV-related periodontal disease

1. HIV infection is increasingly prevalent in the population, and is sometimes associated with marked periodontal destruction.

2. Patients with HIV infection may suffer from an increased prevalence of all types of periodontal disease. In addition, two characteristic periodontal diseases are sometimes seen: HIV-associated gingivitis and HIV-associated periodontitis.

3. HIV-associated gingivitis is characterized by a broad erythematous band affecting both the free and attached gingivae, and is associated with bacteria normally found in subgingival plaque.

4. HIV-associated periodontitis is characterized by periodontitis with superficial necrosis, which clinically may resemble a chronic form of ANUG. This spreads to the deeper tissues causing rapid periodontal breakdown and tooth loss. The microflora is similar to that found in adult periodontitis, but in addition *Candida* has been isolated.

7.6.4 Gingival recession

1. Gingival recession may be caused by periodontal disease, or may result from chronic minor trauma to the gingivae, such as may occur from vigorous scrubbing during toothbrushing.

2. Recession is seen in areas where the alveolar bone and gingiva overlying the tooth are particularly thin, such as on the labial surfaces of lower incisors and upper canine teeth.

3. Recession may be widespread following periodontal treatment, and is due to tissue loss and the shrinkage of tissues during healing.

7.7 Further reading

Baker, D.L. and Seymour, G.J. (1976). The possible pathogenesis of gingival recession in the rat. A histological study of induced recession in the rat. *J. Clin. Periodontol.* **3**, 208–19.
— *One of the few studies investigating the pathogenesis of gingival recession.*

Falkler, W.A. Jr, Martin, S.A., Vincent, J.W., Tall, B.D., Nouman, R.K., and Suzuki, J.B. (1987). A clinical demographic and microbiologic study of ANUG patients in an urban dental school. *J. Clin. Periodont.* **14**, 307–14.

Loesche, W.J., Syed. S.A., Laughton, B.E., and Stoll, J. (1982). The bacteriology of acute necrotizing ulcerative gingivitis. *J. Periodontol.* **53**, 223–30.

Page, R.C. and Schroeder, H.E. (1986). *Periodontitis in man and other animals.* (Karger, Basel).
— *Extensive discussion of the natural history of periodontal disease and classification of the various types of the disease.*

Potter, R.H. (1990). Guest editorial: Genetic studies of juvenile periodontitis. *J. Dent. Res.* **69**, 94–5.
— *A discussion paper on the current status of genetic influences in early onset periodontitis.*

Robertson, P.B. and Greenspan, J.S. (eds). (1988). Perspectives on oral manifestations of AIDS. (PSG Publishing, Littleton, MA).
— *Valuable book on oral aspects of HIV infection, including chapters on HIV-associated periodontal disease.*

Spektor, M.D., Vandesteen, G.E., and Page, R.C. (1985). Clinical studies of one family manifesting rapidly progressive, juvenile and prepubertal periodontitis. *J. Periodontol,* **56**, 93–101.

Watanabe, K. (1990). Pre-pubertal periodontitis: a review of diagnostic criteria, pathogenesis, and differential diagnosis. *J. Periodont. Res.* **25**, 31–48.
— *A useful review of pre-pubertal periodontitis and other causes of periodontal disease in the deciduous dentition.*

Winkler, J.R., Murray, P.A., Grassi, M., and Hammerle, C. (1989). Diagnosis and management of HIV-associated periodontal lesions. *J. Am. Dent. Ass. Supplement.* 25S–34S.
— *Review of HIV-associated periodontal disease.*

8 Clinical management of periodontal disease

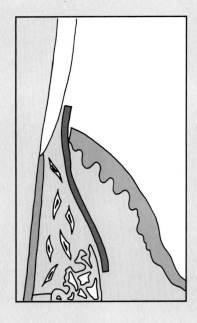

In order to understand the principles of periodontal treatment it is important to have an appreciation of the nature of the disease and its causes. This chapter examines the significance of the pathogenesis of periodontal disease in its clinical management. On pp. 126–7 we discuss the principles and aims of treatment; the methods used to achieve these aims and their rationale are considered on pp. 127–34. Responses to treatment, post-operative healing, and treatment failures are discussed on pp. 134–9. Finally, on pp. 140–1 we discuss some of the developments which may have important consequences for the understanding and management of periodontal disease in the future. This chapter is not intended as an extensive review of the clinical practice of periodontology, for which the reader is referred to one of the excellent texts on the subject.

8.1 Principles of periodontal treatment

8.1.1 General principles

A chronic inflammatory condition is one where there is longstanding inflammation with simultaneous attempts at repair. If the cause of the inflammation is removed, then the condition will resolve. Consequently, the treatment of periodontal disease depends on the elimination of the micro-organisms in plaque from the affected site. Once plaque has been removed, the source of tissue damage is also removed and healing will occur. To a great extent the whole of clinical periodontology revolves around the aim of plaque elimination. Numerous clinical trials have demonstrated that effective periodontal treatment depends principally on effective plaque removal. These studies have shown that patients need to maintain a high level of supragingival plaque control over a long period of time, and that successful treatment also depends on adequate removal of subgingival plaque and calculus by the dentist or hygienist. No single method of treating periodontal disease is predictably more successful than any other method.

8.1.2 Specific aims of treatment

Before specific methods of treatment are considered, it is important to have a clear understanding of their objectives.

Prevention of tooth loss

The principal aim of periodontal treatment is the prevention of tooth loss. As has been noted already, the progression of periodontal disease is not uniform and, at least theoretically, it is only necessary to treat those sites which are likely to progress in the future in order to prevent tooth loss. Additionally, it may also be desirable to prevent further damage and maintain periodontal support.

Maintenance of periodontal support

Even in the absence of tooth loss, damage to the periodontal tissues may have unacceptable sequelae, including increased mobility and drifting of teeth. At present there are no accurate markers that allow the clinician to distinguish between sites which are likely to progress and those which may remain quiescent. Consequently, if the risk of further damage is to be avoided it is necessary to eliminate existing inflammation by removing plaque. Clinical studies demonstrate that inflamed sites will not necessarily deteriorate in the future, although many do progress. In contrast, sites which are not inflamed are very unlikely to break down in the future. In the absence of better predictive markers of future disease progression, the elimination of inflammation is at present the most reliable way of preventing further damage.

In addition to eliminating plaque from the site, periodontal treatment may have secondary aims which help to prevent the disease recurring in the future. These include the treatment of existing periodontal pockets to eliminate the subgingival environment which favours the persistence of pathogenic bacteria (see Chapter 4). This can be achieved either by encouraging the pocket to close up against the root surface, traditionally referred to as 'pocket correction', or by surgically removing all of the tissue making up the pocket, traditionally referred to as 'pocket elimination'.

Repair of damaged tissues and restoration of function

Where the disease has already resulted in significant damage to the tissues, it may be desirable to repair the damaged periodontium in order to restore function. Aims of such treatment include the repair of gingival connective tissue to re-establish a tight cuff around the tooth and the regeneration of alveolar bone and periodontal ligament where these have been lost. The regeneration of the periodontal ligament and associated bone is known as new attachment formation and achievement of this is one of the major challenges in current periodontal therapy. New attachment formation will be considered further on pp. 138–9.

8.2 Methods of treatment

Methods for the treatment of periodontal disease have developed over many years, but until relatively recently many had not been evaluated objectively. Over the last 25 years or so, the effectiveness of different forms of treatment has been tested rigorously and, together with greater understanding of the pathogenesis of periodontal disease, this has led to a sound scientific basis for currently used techniques. Methods of treatment will be considered here under the two sub-headings of supragingival plaque control and subgingival plaque control. Plaque removal is usually carried out by mechanical means, although chemical plaque control can sometimes be a useful adjunct to these methods.

8.2.1 Supragingival plaque control

In Chapter 4 it was shown that, as dental plaque matures, there is an increase in the numbers of organisms which may cause periodontal disease, such as many Gram-negative anaerobic bacteria. Whilst it may not be realistic or necessary to prevent early colonization of teeth by all micro-organisms, regular removal of plaque will prevent the development of a pathogenic flora. In theory at least, complete plaque removal every 48 hours is probably all that is required to prevent the development of periodontal disease. However, this task is extremely difficult to achieve and much greater success is usually achieved by more regular plaque removal. Of course, other considerations of personal hygiene also make more regular cleaning desirable.

Mechanical plaque control

Mechanical plaque control is the cornerstone of periodontal treatment. As it is necessary to carry this out very regularly, it is principally the responsibility of the patient, without whose cooperation treatment will not be successful. Specific techniques of toothbrushing, interdental cleaning, and approaches to patient education are beyond the scope of this book, and are well dealt with elsewhere. Toothpastes contain detergents and mild abrasives which enhance the effectiveness of brushing and result in the removal of bacteria from the tooth surfaces, together with the acquired pellicle which the colonizing bacteria require to adhere to the teeth. The recolonization of bacteria following such cleaning is described in Chapter 4.

In Chapter 1, a number of local aetiological factors were described (see Table 8.1) which can act as mechanical plaque traps, making it difficult or impossible to remove plaque by conventional means. It is the responsibility of the clinician to remove these factors wherever possible to allow effective cleaning by the patient. Supragingival calculus deposits should be removed by scaling as they are too hard to be removed by the patient. Although calculus does not in itself cause periodontal disease, it provides an ideal surface for plaque to colonize and has a layer of viable plaque on its surface. Effective tooth cleaning is not possible without removal of any calculus present.

Table 8.1 Secondary local aetiological factors which may predispose to periodontal disease

Mechanical plaque traps
  Calculus
  Carious cavities
  Margins of restorations
  Partial dentures and other intra-oral appliances
  Crowding and malocclusions
  Anatomical variations of tooth morphology

Decreased anti-bacterial actions of saliva
  Mouthbreathing
  Xerostomia

Occlusal trauma
  Unknown mechanism

Chemical plaque control

For many people, keeping teeth clean enough to prevent or control periodontal disease by oral hygiene measures is both difficult and demanding. There is considerable interest in the use of chemical agents to help control plaque, and some of those that have been proposed are shown in Table 8.2. Antiseptics are active against a wide range of organisms, and resistance is not usually a problem because of their modes of action. For these reasons, the use of antiseptics in toothpastes or mouthwashes to aid supragingival plaque control has been widely investigated.

A number of antiseptics are active against oral bacteria, and some of those have been used as agents for the control of plaque. These include chlorhexidine, hexetidine, cetylpyridium chloride, zinc ions (zinc citrate), triclosan, and sanguinarine. However when evaluating the claims of antiseptics used in dentifrices

Table 8.2 Some chemicals which have been utilized for the control of supragingival plaque

Antiseptics	
Chlorhexidine digluconate	Bisbiguanide. Most effective anti-plaque agent available to date
Povidine iodine	Halogenated compound
Triclosan	Halogenated compound
Cetylpyridium chloride	Quarternary ammonium compound
Benzalkonium chloride	Quarternary ammonium compound
Sanguinarine	Naturally occurring antiseptic obtained from plants
Zinc ions (zinc citrate)	Possible synergistic effects obtained when used with triclosan and hexetidine
Oxidizing agents	
Hydrogen peroxide and sodium perborate	Useful in the management of ANUG
Enzymes	
Glucose oxidase and amyloglucose oxidase	Activates lactoperoxidase system in saliva
Surface active agents	
Octapinol	Sugar alcohol. Acts by inhibiting bacterial colonization of the tooth surface

and mouthwashes it is important to distinguish between the measurable antibacterial effect which can be demonstrated under laboratory conditions and a clinically useful reduction in plaque and inflammation. Many agents which do have antibacterial activity appear to have very limited clinical effects, although some may have benefits when used as an adjunct to mechanical plaque control procedures.

Chlorhexidine digluconate is an extremely effective anti-plaque agent; it is widely used and has been investigated extensively. It is available in the UK as a 0.2 per cent aqueous solution for use as a mouthwash, or as a 1 per cent gel formulation for toothbrushing. It is effective against a very broad range of oral micro-organisms and significant bacterial resistance does not appear to occur, even following long-term use. It is the only available agent which is effective enough to be able to completely replace mechanical toothbrushing. Use of chlorhexidine results in a marked reduction in the number of microorganisms within the oral cavity, with marked inhibition of supragingival plaque formation. It is strongly charged, so that it binds to tooth surfaces and to oral mucosa, retaining the antiseptic activity within the mouth for many hours. This is one of the reasons why it is so effective as an anti-plaque agent, but it also accounts for one of its most troublesome side effects, that of causing staining of the teeth. Unfortunately, this problem is sufficiently severe to limit long term use of chlorhexidine as a general method of controlling plaque. However, it is extremely useful for short-term use, where normal plaque control measures cannot be performed, for example immediately after periodontal surgery.

In addition to antiseptics, a number of other agents have been proposed which may have anti-plaque activity. Oxidizing agents, such as a dilute hydrogen peroxide or sodium perborate solution have been found to be useful in the management of cases of ANUG, but they have little or no effect on other types of periodontal disease. Enzymes which can activate the antibacterial effects of the salivary lactoperoxidase system (described on pp. 69–70) and surface active agents which may inhibit bacterial colonization of the teeth have also been suggested as anti-plaque agents, but require further study. The search for an acceptable and effective method of chemical plaque control continues.

8.2.2 Subgingival plaque control

Where periodontal disease has resulted in the formation of periodontal pockets, the subgingival microflora is largely unaffected by attempts to remove supra-gingival plaque. This is true both for mechanical plaque control methods and antiseptics such as chlorhexidine. Accordingly, it is necessary for the clinician to remove subgingival plaque and calculus, and this can be carried out by non-surgical methods such as scaling and root planing, by open debridement with periodontal surgery, and, on occasions, by the use of adjunctive chemical methods.

Subgingival scaling and root planing

Subgingival scaling is the removal of subgingival plaque and calculus, whilst root planing involves the removal of the surface layers of cementum to eliminate any contamination of the root surface. Although these procedures may have different objectives, in practice they are almost identical and are often simply referred to as deep scaling. Many of the micro-organisms in a pocket are part of the adherent plaque, which is attached to the root surface via a cuticle layer, and cleaning the root surface is therefore generally an effective way of removing them. Subgingival calculus is widely found throughout most periodontal pockets, and is more heavily mineralized than supragingival plaque. It adheres tenaciously to the root surface via the cuticle on the root surface. Whilst there are isolated reports of pockets healing in the presence of residual calculus, it is usually considered essential to remove it all from the root surface to eliminate a potential focus for the colonization and growth of plaque organisms.

The root surface in periodontal disease

Following pocket formation, when the junctional epithelium has migrated apically and the cementum has become exposed to the pocket environment, the root surface undergoes a number of changes which influence periodontal treatment (Table 8.3). First, the cementoblast layer on the root surface is lost and the cementum becomes devitalized. The root surface becomes coated by a cuticle layer due to the adsorption of proteins from crevicular fluid, and this layer may become mineralized. The root surface is colonized by bacteria which adhere to the cuticle, and physico-chemical alterations occur, such as the surface layer of cementum becoming hypermineralized. The cementum also becomes contaminated by pathogenic bacterial products, particularly endotoxins, and it

---

Table 8.3   Alterations to the root surface after pocket formation

Loss of cementoblast layer and cementum vitality
Hypermineralization of the superficial cementum
Formation of a cuticle layer
Colonization of the root surface by plaque and calculus
Adsorption of bacterial virulence factors (e.g. endotoxin) to root surface
Presence of isolated resorption lacunae

has been suggested that it is necessary to remove extensive amounts of cementum by root planing in order to eliminate absorbed endotoxin. Recent evidence has shown that contamination of cementum is restricted to adsorption of material on to the superficial layers of the root surface, and that extensive removal of cementum by root planing is not necessary for the removal of endotoxins and other bacterial products (see Fig. 8.1). Thus it appears that the main benefits of the removal of the superficial cementum by root planing are that it facilitates the elimination of plaque and calculus from irregularities present on the root surface, such as those made by isolated resorption lacunae (see Fig. 8.2).

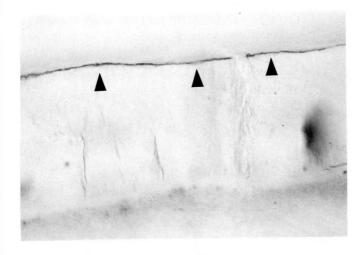

Fig. 8.1 Detail of ground section of cementum exposed to a periodontal pocket, stained for endotoxins using labelled antibodies. Endotoxins are confined to the cementum surface (arrows) as shown by the surface staining (magnification × 160).

The efficacy of subgingival scaling

A number of studies have demonstrated that it is virtually impossible to eliminate plaque bacteria entirely from the pocket by subgingival scaling, particularly where the bacteria are deep. In addition, the procedure is very likely to introduce bacteria into the gingival tissues from the pocket environment. Nevertheless, clinical studies show that such treatment is generally effective in the treatment of periodontal disease. The reasons for this are that the procedure results in marked changes in the composition of the flora and that residual bacteria are more readily eliminated by host defences once the main bulk of plaque is removed.

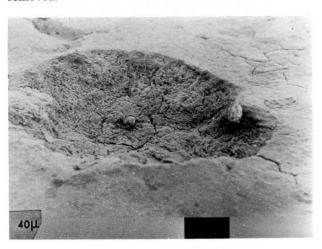

Fig. 8.2 Scanning electron micrograph of an isolated resorption lacuna on a root surface exposed to a periodontal pocket.

Periodontal surgery

The main limitation of non-surgical techniques for subgingival plaque control is the technical difficulty of cleaning the root surface without direct vision. Although surgical techniques do not have a consistent advantage over non-surgical techniques in the treatment of periodontal pocketing, there are times when it may be preferable to utilize a surgical approach. This is particularly the case where pockets have failed to repond to earlier treatment, or where access for non-surgical treatment is poor. Periodontal surgery involves raising a soft tissue flap in order to gain direct access to the root surface, allowing subgingival debridement to be carried out with direct vision. The inverse bevel flap procedure has been widely used and evaluated as an effective surgical procedure. This procedure involves the excision of the pocket lining and the lifting of a muco-periosteal flap to expose the affected root surfaces (see Fig. 8.3). With the flap

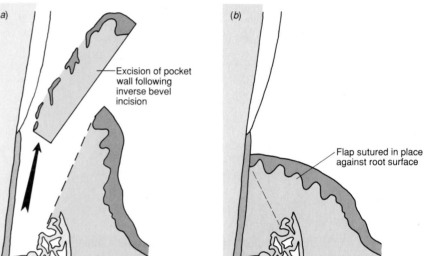

Fig. 8.3 The inverse bevel flap.

(a) The soft tissue pocket wall is excised by making an incision from the gingival margin to the crestal bone at an angle of about 10° to the long axis of the tooth. This tissue is then removed and the flap is elevated to expose the root surface.

(b) Immediately after debridement, the flap is replaced against the root surface and sutured in place. Some recession may result from the removal of tissue.

(a) — Excision of pocket wall following inverse bevel incision

(b) — Flap sutured in place against root surface

elevated, the root surface is cleaned under direct vision by scaling and root planing. In the past, much emphasis has been placed on the importance of removal of granulation tissue during periodontal surgery to eliminate inflammation and bacteria which were thought to be in the tissue. However, as the formation of granulation tissue is a reflection of attempted healing at a chronically inflamed site, there seems little merit in the removal of granulation tissue unless it obscures direct vision during debridement of the root surface. Finally, if connective tissue attachment and periodontal regeneration is to occur (see pp. 138–9), then it is necessary to remove the epithelial lining of the pocket wall to allow the connective tissue to contact the root surface.

Chemical control of subgingival plaque

Topical antimicrobial chemotherapy

The main factor which influences the effectiveness of topical chemical agents in the control of subgingival plaque is achieving a high enough concentration in the pocket for a sufficient period of time. Many of the antiseptic agents described for supragingival plaque control have been used subgingivally and, in addition, antibiotics have been used. Agents which are applied supragingivally do not penetrate into the pocket, and the irrigation of pockets by agents such as chlorhexidine has been advocated and is widely utilized following subgingival scaling. Unfortunately, clinical trials have not demonstrated any clear advantages of this technique when compared with the effects of subgingival scaling alone.

To overcome the problems of keeping chemotherapeutic agents in the pocket for long enough to be effective, materials which can be placed directly into a pocket and which release the agent slowly have been developed. Such devices, known as slow release delivery systems, have utilized a number of different agents, including chlorhexidine, tetracycline, and metronidazole. The delivery sytems include acrylic strips impregnated with the drug, dialysis tubing containing the drug, and fibres made of synthetic polymers. They are placed in the periodontal pocket and have to be removed at a later date. Their advantage is that it is possible to obtain high doses of the active agent at the site where it is required, whilst at the same time avoiding significant levels throughout the rest of the body. This minimizes side effects and reduces the development of drug resistance in the patient's normal flora at other sites. These systems are still under development, but show promise as adjuncts to conventional methods of subgingival plaque control.

Systemic antimicrobial chemotherapy

Unlike antiseptics, antibiotics have more specific modes of action and a narrower spectrum of activity. As a result, they are suitable for systemic administration and can be chosen to be selective for specific target micro-organisms. In periodontal disease, the choice of antibiotic is influenced by current thinking on the nature of periodontal pathogens, but may also be based on microbiological culture and antibiotic sensitivity testing for individual affected sites. Theoretically it should be possible to use an antibiotic which eliminates pathogenic bacteria without affecting other commensals, resulting in a shift from a pathogenic to a non-pathogenic plaque. However, the use of antibiotics cannot be regarded as a substitute for effective mechanical plaque control, because if antibiotic treatment alone is used the changes in the flora are only transient and periodontal pathogens rapidly recolonize the pocket. There is little or no benefit to be gained from the routine use of antibiotics as an adjunct to conventional treatment, because mechanical treatments are generally equally effective on their own. In a few special cases, such as patients with early onset periodontitis or refractory periodontitis, adjunctive antibiotic therapy is a valuable tool in the treatment of disease. Two antibiotics in particular have been used extensively for treatment of these conditions: tetracycline – and related drugs such as minocycline and doxycycline – and metronidazole.

Tetracycline is a broad spectrum bacteriostatic antibiotic effective against nearly all oral organisms, including *A. actinomycetemcomitans* and *P. gingivalis*. It is unusual in that it is found in crevicular fluid at considerably higher concentrations than the circulating serum concentrations following its systemic administration. It has also been found to inhibit the activity of some collagenase enzymes, which could help to decrease tissue destruction in periodontal disease. The importance of this observation has yet to be determined. Tetracycline has been used with considerable success in cases of early onset periodontitis and refractory adult periodontitis.

Metronidazole has a narrower spectrum of activity than tetracycline, being active against obligate anaerobic organisms. It is active against most periodontal pathogens, including *P. gingivalis*, but *A. actinomycetemcomitans* is often resistant to it. Metronidazole is of value in the treatment of refractory adult periodontitis and in cases of rapidly progressive periodontitis, but is not particularly useful in the treatment of localized juvenile periodontitis. It is extremely effective in cases of acute necrotizing ulcerative gingivitis, and in HIV-related periodontal disease. Metronidazole has also been used in combination with amoxycillin, which increases the spectrum of organisms which are susceptible and reduces problems of bacterial resistance. However, this combination of drugs is often used in the treatment of serious and life-threatening infections, and it is not justified to use it for the management of periodontal disease. A summary of the uses of systemic antibiotics in the management of periodontal disease is given in Table 8.4.

Table 8.4 Potential uses of antibiotics in the treatment of periodontal disease

Indication	Drug	Dose
Management of acute periodontal abscesses	Penicillin V *or* Metronidazole	250–500 mg QDS. 7 days 200 mg TDS. 7 days
Severe ANUG/HIV-associated periodontitis	Metronidazole *or* Penicillin V	200 mg TDS. 3 days 250 mg QDS. 5 days (longer in HIV infection)
Early onset periodontitis (concurrent with mechanical debridement)	Tetracycline	250 mg QDS. 3 weeks
Refractory adult periodontitis (concurrent with mechanical debridement)	Tetracycline *or* Metronidazole	250 mg QDS. 3 weeks 200 mg TDS. 2 weeks

In addition antibiotics are used for prophylaxis against infective endocarditis prior to periodontal treatment.

8.3 Responses to treatment

8.3.1 The effects of treatment

Effects of mechanical plaque control on the microflora

Although plaque control procedures appear to have a very broad and unsophisticated objective of reducing the total number of organisms present, the alterations in the flora following plaque removal are actually more complex and subtle than might at first be thought. Following complete plaque removal, there is a radical alteration in the predominant flora. In addition to a marked reduction in the total number of organisms, the proportion of Gram-negative anaerobic organisms is greatly reduced, the residual flora being predominantly Gram-positive and aerobic. The composition of the flora changes from that which is generally associated with diseased sites towards one which is generally associated with health. This is a good illustration of how one balanced ecosystem within the pocket can be disrupted and replaced with another which is ecologically stable, but is not damaging. These qualitative changes in the subgingival flora are partly due to a reduction in plaque thickness, which leads to effects such as a higher oxygen concentration within the plaque. The reduction in the variety of bacterial species makes it difficult for the more fastidious Gram-negative anaerobes to become re-established in the flora. The reduction in the mass of plaque also renders residual organisms in the pocket more susceptible to neutralization and killing by host defence mechanisms operating in the pocket.

If the new flora is stable and supragingival plaque is controlled, anaerobic Gram-negative organisms are less likely to re-colonize the pocket, and healing will take place.

Healing of the periodontal tissues

The general features and regulation of postoperative healing of the periodontal tissues are essentially the same as that seen for any chronically inflamed site. Following debridement there is an initial acute inflammatory reaction as the result of the trauma from the treatment itself, but within 24–48 hours the inflammation begins to subside. Over the next week there is a gradual reduction in vasodilation, crevicular fluid flow, and the number of inflammatory cells; ulcers present in the pocket epithelium also begin to heal. Fibroblasts migrate towards the inflamed tissues and proliferate, and collagen fibres and ground substance are laid down (Fig. 8.4(b)). Over a period of a few weeks the connective tissue matures with the deposition of fibrous tissue organized in the same way as in health (Fig. 8.4(c)). In contrast, relatively little bony healing takes place in the alveolar bone, with only a limited amount of re-modelling at the alveolar crest being evident.

The pocket epithelium begins to re-attach to the root surface, with the formation of a basement membrane and hemidesmosomes which attach the keratinocytes to the cementum. This is referred to as the formation of a long epithelial attachment or long junctional epithelium. The formation of a long epithelial attachment results in the gradual closure of the pocket, and may continue for some months after treatment (Fig. 8.4(d)). The clinical changes observed during healing are the result of these the changes in the tissues. Initially, there is a reduction in redness and swelling as the inflammation subsides. Bleeding on probing is also reduced as the inflammation subsides and ulcers in the pocket epithelium heal. The gingivae become increasingly pink and firm in appearance as the connective tissue matures. The reduction in probing depth associated with periodontal healing is the result of shrinkage of the tissues as inflammation subsides, a tightening of the gingival cuff formed by the orientation of the healthy gingival collagen fibres, and formation of the long epithelial attachment.

The events which occur following periodontal surgery are essentially the same as those described above, but where the pocket epithelium has been excised the oral epithelium at the edge of the surgical wound proliferates and cells migrate apically to form a new pocket epithelium and junctional epithelium. This process probably only takes a few days to occur. Previously, it was thought that the excision of the pocket epithelium would promote new connective tissue attachment to the root surface, but it is now known that this does not usually occur, although a small amount of new attachment formation may occur at the most apical extent of the pocket. Thus the epithelium will eventually form a long epithelial attachment in exactly the same way as is seen following non-surgical treatment.

The regulation of healing

Healing occurs partly because the elimination of inflammation allows the restoration of normal regulatory mechanisms of tissue homeostasis described in Chapter 2, and partly because of specific factors which promote healing following treatment. These have already been discussed on pp. 102–3, but they will be reviewed briefly here. Cytokines are known to be released during healing, and are thought to have important regulatory functions, but other regulatory

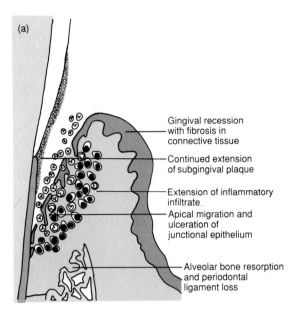

Gingival recession with fibrosis in connective tissue

Continued extension of subgingival plaque

Extension of inflammatory infiltrate

Apical migration and ulceration of junctional epithelium

Alveolar bone resorption and periodontal ligament loss

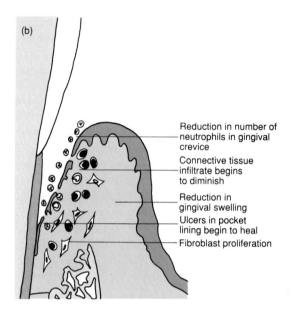

Reduction in number of neutrophils in gingival crevice

Connective tissue infiltrate begins to diminish

Reduction in gingival swelling

Ulcers in pocket lining begin to heal

Fibroblast proliferation

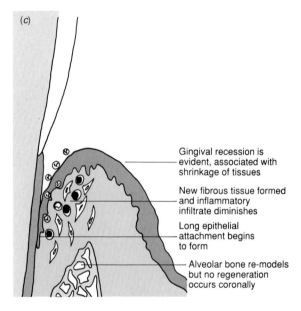

Gingival recession is evident, associated with shrinkage of tissues

New fibrous tissue formed and inflammatory infiltrate diminishes

Long epithelial attachment begins to form

Alveolar bone re-models but no regeneration occurs coronally

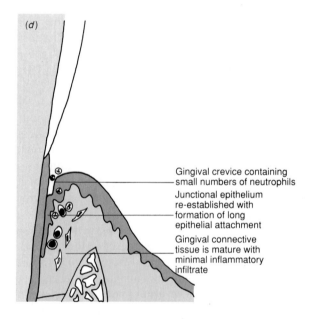

Gingival crevice containing small numbers of neutrophils

Junctional epithelium re-established with formation of long epithelial attachment

Gingival connective tissue is mature with minimal inflammatory infiltrate

Fig. 8.4 Stages of healing of a periodontal pocket. The time-scale given is only an approximation and may vary considerably).

(a) Prior to treatment. The advanced lesion, as previously described in Chapter 3.

(b) One week post treatment. Following plaque removal, inflammation begins to subside. There is a gradual reduction in exudate and numbers of inflammatory cells. Ulcers in the pocket epithelium heal. Fibroblasts and endothelial cells migrate into and proliferate in the previously inflamed areas. Clinically, there is reduction in swelling and redness of the gingivae.

(c) One month post treatment. Inflammation has subsided and new gingival connective tissue

is laid down. The alveolar crestal bone is re-modelled, but does not regenerate coronally. Long epithelial attachment formation is evident at the most apical extent of the pocket. Clinically, there is a reduction in bleeding on probing and reduced pocket depths; some recession may be evident due to shrinkage of tissues.

(d) 3–6 months post treatment. A fully healed periodontal pocket. Long epithelial attachment formation is complete and there is mature gingival connective tissue. Clinically, the site does not bleed on probing and pocket depths are reduced to within physiological limits.

mechanisms such as direct cell contacts and interactions with matrix molecules are probably also important.

Proliferation and healing of the ulcerated pocket is stimulated by cytokines such as TGFα, and once epithelial continuity is restored it is then inhibited by contact inhibition or cytokines such as TGFβ. Epithelial cell attachment is promoted by basement membrane proteins such as laminin. Fibroblasts are attracted into damaged tissue chemotactically by factors such as TGFβ and platelet derived growth factor (PDGF) and matrix synthesis is stimulated by TGFβ. Fibroblasts are also regulated by interactions with matrix components, such as proteoglycans, and cell attachment molecules like fibronectin and tenascin, resulting in stimulation of matrix synthesis, proliferation, and tissue morphogenesis. The precise importance of any one of these mechanisms remains to be determined.

8.3.2 Treatment failures

Common causes of treatment failures

On some occasions, healing does not progress and the pocket fails to respond to treatment, as determined by the continued presence of inflammation and the lack of reduction in pocket depths. Most treatment failures occur either because the root surface was not adequately cleaned during treatment, or because the site has not been kept free of supragingival plaque. In both instances, the subgingival flora becomes re-established rapidly, resulting in the continuation of inflammation, and the failure of the pocket to heal. Where oral hygiene measures are not maintained adequately after treatment, supragingival plaque rapidly reforms and matures and subgingival plaque reforms as a result of apical extension of the supragingival plaque. Within a few weeks the subgingival flora has a similar composition to that found prior to treatment.

Refractory periodontitis

In a few cases, patients do not respond well to treatment even though plaque control has remained optimal and the root surface has been adequately cleaned. These cases are refractory to normal methods of treatment and are sometimes referred to as refractory periodontitis. Many cases of early onset periodontitis appear to be unusually resistant to normal treatment regimens, but in addition there may be up to 10 per cent of cases of adult periodontitis which fall into this category. It is not clear why some cases should be more resistant to treatment. Current investigations into the aetiology of refractory cases have focused on microbiological studies, although refractory periodontitis may sometimes be associated with impaired neutrophil function.

Following treatment, there is a marked change in the composition of the subgingival flora, with the disappearance of periodontal pathogens. Studies have shown that *P. gingivalis*, for example, can be eliminated from subgingival plaque in over 80 per cent of cases following deep scaling. However, this is far less effective in eliminating *A. actinomycetemcomitans* from the flora, which persists in over 50 per cent of cases after treatment. Current evidence suggests that refractory periodontitis is associated with the persistence of pathogenic bacteria in the pocket following treatment. This is supported by studies which have treated early onset and refractory periodontitis successfully using adjunctive antibiotic therapy. However, it is not clear whether refractory periodontitis is caused by the presence of bacteria, such as *A. actinomycetemcomitans*, which are difficult to remove by conventional treatment, or if the persistence of pathogenic bacteria is the result of other factors such as temporary host defence defects.

8.3.3 New attachment formation

Principles of new attachment formation

Whilst periodontal treatment is generally effective in preventing further periodontal destruction, regeneration of the periodontal tissues does not usually result. Although healing by formation of a long epithelial attachment is effective in preventing tooth loss, complete regeneration of the periodontal tissues is a desirable aim, particularly where gross periodontal destruction has compromized the support of the affected tooth. This requires the attachment of periodontal ligament cells and fibres to the previously denuded root surface with new cementum formation, the formation of a functionally orientated fibre network emanating from the root, and the coronal regrowth of the alveolar bone. It has long been the aim of periodontists to find treatment procedures which would promote periodontal regeneration (new attachment). However, limited new attachment formation or bone regeneration is only rarely seen, and then usually only in the depths of infrabony pockets.

It is clear that bone and fibrous tissues have the potential for regeneration, as evidenced by wound healing in other parts of the body. The reasons why new attachment formation does not occur following periodontal treatment are not fully understood, but may be related to the requirements for new attachment formation to take place. These include the exclusion of epithelium from the wound area, the adequate debridement of the root surface, and the repopulation of the site by appropriate progenitor cells to form periodontal ligament. The presence of the epithelium between the connective tissue and the root surface will prevent fibroblasts becoming attached to the cementum and will inhibit new attachment formation. Root surface debridement is important in providing a suitable surface for cells to attach to, and wound repopulation by appropriate cells is necessary if new bone, cementum, and periodontal ligament are to form.

It is possible that periodontal ligament cells are unique in their ability to form new attachment. It has been suggested that the cells of the periodontal ligament can regenerate from a common progenitor cell which is able to differentiate into fibroblasts, cementoblasts, or osteoblasts, as happens in the dental follicle during tooth development. Alternatively, progenitor cells from endosteal spaces migrate into the periodontal ligament.

The main techniques that have been proposed to promote new attachment formation include bone grafting, the conditioning of root surfaces by demineralization, and the use of membranes to regulate the types of cells participating in the healing process. The latter technique is known as guided tissue regeneration. A variety of different bone graft materials have been tested for their ability to stimulate new attachment formation by promoting the regrowth of crestal alveolar bone. These include autógenous bone chips obtained from the patient's iliac crest, and artificial hydroxyapatite implants. Bone graft materials could act in a number of ways, but they act principally as a framework for osteoblasts to colonize and deposit new bone. In addition, bone matrix contains a number of growth factors which might be released to promote bone formation. Whilst there have been anecdotal reports of the use of such techniques, there are relatively few properly controlled studies which demonstrate their efficacy or show new attachment formation as a result of their use. The histological evidence suggests that on many occasions the grafts are not replaced by new bone, but are encapsulated in fibrous tissue without any evidence of true periodontal ligament regeneration *per se*. Furthermore, it has not been convincingly demonstrated that new bone formation at the alveolar crest will lead to new periodontal ligament formation, which is one of the fundamental assumptions in the use of these techniques.

Another technique which has attracted some interest is the surface demineralization of the root surface using citric acid. This procedure has a number of effects, including the exposure of unmineralized collagen fibrils which promote attachment by fibroblasts and allow new collagen fibres to be spliced onto them. The promotion of fibroblast attachment may also have the secondary effect of inhibiting epithelial cell downgrowth. However, clinical results with this technique have been disappointing, despite early encouraging results from animal studies.

Guided tissue regeneration

At present, the most successful method of promoting new attachment formation is the technique of guided tissue regeneration. This involves the use of a mechanical barrier to determine which cells repopulate the wound following periodontal surgery. After removal of the pocket lining and thorough debridement of the site, a membrane is interposed between the flap and the root surface before suturing (Fig. 8.5). This effectively excludes the epithelium and gingival connective tissue from the root surface during healing, and promotes repopulation by cells derived from the periodontal ligament and bone. Membranes made from polytetrafluoroethylene (PTFE, teflon) fibres are commercially available, although other materials have been used successfully. After about six weeks, the membrane is removed by a second surgical procedure. Guided tissue regeneration has recently become widely used, particularly for the treatment of furcation defects and in infrabony pockets, where it appears to be particularly effective. Long-term evaluation of the results of this procedure remains to be fully established, but it appears to represent a major advance in attempts to promote new attachment formation following periodontal treatment.

Fig. 8.5 Principles of guided tissue regeneration.
  (a) The pocket epithelium is excised and the root surface debrided in the same way as for the conventional inverse bevel flap procedure.

  (b) Before replacing the flap, a membrane is interposed between the flap and the root surface. The membrane excludes the epithelium and gingival connective tissue from the healing wound, and promotes repopulation by cells migrating from the periodontal ligament below.

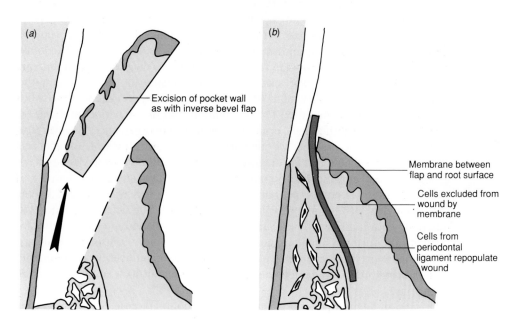

(a)

Excision of pocket wall as with inverse bevel flap

(b)

Membrane between flap and root surface

Cells excluded from wound by membrane

Cells from periodontal ligament repopulate wound

8.4 Future prospects for the management of periodontal disease

In this section, some future developments in the management of periodontal disease are considered. These prospects include better methods of preventing disease, better diagnostic tests, improved chemotherapy, and methods for rgeliable new attachment formation. This is not, of course, a comprehensive list, but highlights some areas where progress is being made.

8.4.1 Prevention of disease

Approaches to the improvement of the periodontal health of the community are largely dependent on improving oral hygiene practices. Whilst there is evidence of improvements in the level of plaque control and overall periodontal health in the community, there is little information as to how such general improvements affect those people who are most at risk from destructive periodontal disease. Information on factors which determine susceptibility to periodontal disease would enable more careful targeting of resources to those most at risk from the disease. A group of patients identified to be at risk from severe periodontal disease might benefit from more regular dental attendance, disease screening, and advice than may be required for the average patient, and it is important that such individuals are recognized at a stage when effective preventive care can be instituted.

8.4.2 Diagnostic testing

There is a need for improved tests for the assessment and diagnosis of patients with periodontal disease, and current research is directed towards finding specific tests for this purpose. These tests would potentially have a number of valuable clinical functions, including the identification of susceptible individuals, the ability to assess effectiveness of treatment and identify refractory cases requiring antimicrobial chemotherapy more accurately, and the ability to identify periods of active periodontal breakdown. For such tests to be of value they should be both sensitive and specific; that is, they should be capable of detecting susceptible patients and of discriminating between these and resistant patients. The kinds of test which are currently being evaluated to improve diagnosis and treatment include the identification of specific micro-organisms in the flora and the measurement of a variety of host factors present in crevicular fluid. Microbiological testing is based on the observation that active periodontal disease is often associated with specific organisms or groups of organisms. However, the identification of the presence of one particular organism has not, so far, been shown to be a reliable test for diagnostic purposes, although test kits based on gene probes and enzyme detection are commercially available.

Tests of host factors for periodontal diagnosis are less well advanced than microbiological testing at present, but include tests for defects in leucocyte function, serum antibody levels, and measurement of factors released into crevicular fluid during tissue damage. Many of the currently utilized methods are too complex or expensive for routine use, but the identification of a suitable marker would probably be followed by its development as a simplified test for clinical use.

In view of the multifactorial aetiology of periodontal disease, it is unlikely that any single test will turn out to be a reliable marker for diagnostic testing, and a combination of tests may be required to improve clinical diagnosis and prognosis.

8.4.3 Chemotherapy

A cheap, safe and effective anti-plaque agent, without significant side effects, might result in a considerable improvement in general periodontal health. The example of the effect of fluoride in toothpastes, which has been associated with a considerable reduction of the prevalence of dental caries in the population, presents the challenge of developing a similar strategy for the reduction of periodontal disease. It remains to be established whether such an effect would be useful in those most at risk from destructive disease.

Slow release delivery systems for the application of antibiotics are already being evaluated in research studies and may become widely used in the future. It is difficult to predict further developments, but there is potential for the use of narrow spectrum chemotherapy specifically directed at bacterial pathogens identified during diagnostic testing. Such agents might be intended to eliminate the offending organisms without substantially changing the rest of the flora.

8.4.4 New attachment

The technique of guided tissue regeneration is already having a great impact on attempts to manipulate healing to gain new attachment. However, the technique is probably not the answer to all the problems of new attachment formation, and its long term effects on alveolar bone regeneration, for example, remain unknown. Research is being conducted into the possibility of using bio-degradeable membranes for guided tissue regeneration, which would obviate the need to carry out the second surgical procedure to recover the membrane. Other experimental approaches towards promoting new attachment include the use of growth factors and other signal molecules to control the behaviour of cells in the healing wound. Studies which have used the attachment factor fibronectin to attempt to promote fibroblast attachment to cementum have been disappointing, although pilot studies using growth factors appear more encouraging. The cost of using purified growth factors makes it unlikely that this will become a routine treatment, but such studies may also provide valuable information about the basic mechanisms of regulation of periodontal wound healing which may be valuable in other ways.

8.5 Summary

1. The treatment of periodontal disease depends on the elimination of its cause. Once plaque is removed, the condition will resolve.

2. The overall aims of periodontal treatment are to arrest periodontal breakdown and to prevent tooth loss. In addition, the restoration of function to damaged tissues is also desirable.

3. Plaque removal is normally achieved by mechanical methods, including effective toothbrushing and subgingival debridement.

4. Topical and systemic antibacterial chemotherapy can be useful adjuncts to

mechanical plaque control in some circumstances, but are not a substitute for them.

5. Plaque removal results in a change in the type of flora remaining as well as the total number of organisms present. Following subgingival debridement there is a marked reduction in the proportion of Gram-negative anaerobic organisms present.

6. The features of periodontal healing include the elimination of inflammation, formation of a fibrous tissue cuff in the gingiva, and closure of the pocket by the formation of a long epithelial attachment.

7. Refractory periodontitis is often associated with the persistence of bacterial pathogens in the pocket. It may respond to adjunctive antibiotic therapy.

8. Guided tissue regeneration uses a mechanical barrier to control the cell types repopulating the healing site and shows promise as a method for promoting new attachment.

9. The prospect of diagnostic tests to identify disease susceptibility and prognosis offers considerable hope for the future if suitable disease markers can be identified.

8.6 Further reading

Lindhe, J. (1987). *A textbook of clinical periodontology* (2nd edn). (Munksgaard, Copenhagen).
— *Comprehensive textbook of periodontology.*

Kieser, J.B. (1990). *Periodontics: a practical approach.* (Wright, London).
— *Up to date textbook of clinical periodontology.*

Rateitschak, K.H., Rateitschak, E.M., Wolf, H.F., and Hassell, T.M. (1989). *A colour atlas of dental medicine 1. Periodontology* (2nd edn). (Thieme, Stuttgart).
— *Well illustrated colour atlas covering all aspects of periodontal treatment.*

Axelsson, P. and Lindhe, J. (1981). The significance of maintenance care in the treatment of periodontal disease. *J. Clin. Periodontol.* **8**, 281–94.

Badersten, A., Nilvéus, R., and Egelberg, J. (1984). Effect of nonsurgical periodontal therapy II. Severely advanced periodontitis. *J. Clin. Periodontol.* **11**, 63–76.

Hill, R.W., Ramfjord, S.P., Morrison, E.C., Appleberry, E.A., Caffesse, R.G., Kerry, G.J., and Nissle, R.R. (1981). Four types of periodontal treatment compared over two years. *J. Periodontol.* **52**, 655–62.

Pihlstrom, B.L., McHugh, R.B., Oliphant, T.H., and Ortiz Campos, C. (1983). Comparison of surgical and nonsurgical treatment of periodontal disease. A review of current studies and additional results after $6\frac{1}{2}$ years. *J. Clin. Periodontol.* **10**, 524–41.
— *Examples of four clinical trials which have had a major impact on current treatment techniques and which emphasize the importance of plaque control over other methods of treatment.*

Gottlow, J., Nyman, S., Karring, T., and Lindhe, J. (1984). New attachment formation as the result of controlled tissue regeneration. *J. Clin. Periodontol.* **11**, 494–503.
— *Description of guided tissue regeneration.*

Joyston Bechal, S. (1987). Topical and systemic antimicrobial agents in the treatment of chronic gingivitis and periodontitis. *Int. Dent. J.* **37**, 52–62.
— *Review of use of chemotherapy in periodontal treatment.*

Listgarten, M. (1986). A persective on periodontal diagnosis. *J. Clin. Periodontol.* **13**, 175–81.
— *Discussion of diagnostic testing.*

Glossary

aetiology
: The cause of a disease, in the case of gingivitis and periodontal disease, microbial dental plaque.

adjuvant
: A non-specific stimulant of the immune response which enhances the response to antigen. Many bacterial cell wall components have this property.

aerobe
: A micro-organism which grows in the presence of oxygen.

anaerobe
: A micro-organism which grows in the absence of oxygen. In practice, most anaerobes are also killed by oxygen (*see also* facultative anaerobe).

anaerobic
: Without oxygen.

antibody
: An immunoglobulin which binds to a specific antigen. Lymphocytes which have recognized an antigen may differentiate into plasma cells and secrete antibody against that antigen.

antigen
: A structure recognized as foreign by the immune system. The word is derived from **anti**body **gen**erator.

bacterial succession
: The appearance and disappearance of species as a mixed flora evolves. An example in plaque is the increase in filamentous bacteria which take over from coccal bacteria as plaque matures. Succession occurs in a predictable sequence as the plaque environment gradually changes to favour different species.

bystander damage
: Accidental damage to host tissues caused by complement, neutrophils, and macrophages during inflammation.

capnophilic
: Bacteria which require carbon dioxide for growth are capnophilic.

chemotaxis
: Locomotion of cells which is directed along an increasing chemical gradient of a soluble substance.

contact inhibition
: Inhibition of movement and division caused by physical contact between cells of the same type.

cytokine

A small protein messenger released by cells which affects the division, differentiation, and function of other cells, which may be of the same or different types. (*See also* lymphokine *and* interleukin.)

desmosome

A specialized attachment between epithelial cells which imparts strength to epithelium.

ecological niche

The functional position which a bacterial species occupies within a complex ecosystem such as plaque. The term does not relate to the physical position of the organism, either on the tooth surface or in plaque.

endotoxin

A complex heat stable toxin which is a structural component of Gram-negative bacterial cell walls. The active component is a lipopolysaccharide.

facultative anaerobe

A micro-organism which, although anaerobic, can survive and grow in the presence of oxygen.

fibronectin

A connective tissue protein which binds cells to the extracellular matrix.

fimbria

A fine filamentous surface appendage on a bacterium. These are important for attachment and adhesion and are important antigens on some species.

F_c

The part of an immunoglobulin molecule which binds to specific receptors on neutrophils and macrophages, but which does not bind to antigen.

glycosaminoglycan

A molecule of repeating sugar subunits which forms a major component of connective tissue ground substance.

gnotobiotic animal

A laboratory animal whose microbial flora is known. Specific microorganisms are introduced into germ-free animals to make them gnotobiotic.

hemidesmosome

Structure which attaches epithelial cells to the basement membrane. It resembles half a desmosome, but has different structural components.

homeostasis

The production of a stable equilibrium in a body system by means of feedback mechanisms.

hydrolytic enzyme

A class of enzymes which cleave various types of bonds, including peptide, ester, and glycosidic bonds, with the addition of water. Many degradative and lysosomal enzymes fall into this category.

immune complex	A complex of antigen and antibody molecules bound to one another and together.
interleukins	Cytokines which mediate communication between leucocytes.
lipopolysaccharide	The active component of bacterial endotoxins.
lymphokine	Cytokines secreted by lymphocytes. Cytokines is now the preferred term for this group of substances because they are secreted by other cell types as well.
metalloproteinases	Enzymes which degrade proteins in the presence of metal ions, usually calcium or magnesium. Many enzymes which degrade connective tissue components are metalloproteinases.
monocyte	A large mononuclear phagocytic leucocyte, the circulating precursors of macrophages.
neutrophil	A phagocytic polymorphonuclear leucocyte.
osteoclast activating factor (OAF)	A mixture of cytokines, including Il-1, TNF, TGFβ, and PDGF, which induces bone resorption and was previously thought to be a distinct cytokine.
opsonin	A substance which facilitates phagocytosis when bound to the surface of a bacterium or other particle.
pathogenesis	The mechanisms by which a disease develops.
pellicle	The earliest layer of plaque composed of salivary glycoprotein, which is later colonized by bacteria.
phagocytosis	The process by which cells internalize particles into an intracellular vacuole.
plaque	A complex mass comprising bacteria, their products, host-derived material, and food debris which adheres to teeth.
plasma cell	A mature B lymphocyte which secretes antibody.
proteoglycan	A protein with numerous glycosaminoglycan side chains. A major component of connective tissue ground substance.
redox potential	A measure of the ease with which oxidation and reduction reactions will occur. Environments which are anaerobic or contain reducing agents, such as periodontal pockets, have a low redox potential.

saccharolytic   Bacteria which break down carbohydrates for
                                       energy are saccharolytic.

synergy   An interaction which is cooperative.

tissue inhibitor of   An enzyme inhibitor secreted by fibroblasts to
metalloproteinases (TIMP)   control the activity of metalloproteinases in the
                                       turnover of connective tissue ground substance.

Index